Weathering the Storm

Leading Your Organization Through a Pandemic

Stephen Prior, Robert Armstrong, and Ford Rowan with Mary Beth Hill-Harmon

Center for Technology and National Security Policy

National Defense University

November 2006

Dr. Stephen Prior is the President of Quantum Leap Health Sciences in Arlington, VA and the Executive Director of the National Center for Critical Incident Analysis in Washington, DC. Dr. Prior is a Distinguished Research Fellow at the Center for Technology and National Security Policy (CTNSP) at the National Defense University (NDU) in Washington, DC. His research interests include the impact of life sciences on military operations and national security and innovative technology for military use. He holds a doctorate in microbial physiology from Warwick University (UK).

Dr. Robert Armstrong is a Senior Research Fellow with the National Defense University's Center for Technology and National Security Policy. He served as a Life Sciences Intelligence Officer with the Central Intelligence Agency and held a senior executive position at the U.S. Department of Agriculture prior to joining the National Defense University. A veteran of Vietnam, he continues to serve as a colonel in the Army Reserve. He holds a doctorate in plant genetics from Purdue University.

Dr. Ford Rowan chairs the National Center for Critical Incident Analysis, an independent research center affiliated with the National Defense University Foundation. He is a lawyer, management consultant and former NBC News national security affairs correspondent. He earned a law degree from Georgetown University and a doctorate in public administration from the University of Southern California.

Mary Beth Hill-Harmon has a MSPH in epidemiology from the Rollins School of Public Health at Emory University. Her work experiences in public health range from working at the Occupational Safety and Health Administration (OSHA) on environmental tobacco smoke standards to being a cancer epidemiologist at the American Cancer Society, where she produced annual facts and figures for the Society's publications. Currently, Ms. Hill-Harmon is a Research Associate at the Center for Technology and National Security Policy.

Defense & Technology Papers are published by the National Defense University Center for Technology and National Security Policy, Fort Lesley J. McNair, Washington, DC. CTNSP publications are available online at http://www.ndu.edu/ctnsp/publications.html.

Contents

Executive Summary

The Calm Before the Storm

A storm is coming. None of us have ever experienced a storm like this. It could arrive very soon. But, as anyone who makes a living as a forecaster will quickly say, "On the other hand . . ."

The storm is, of course, an influenza pandemic. Much has been written in the past few years about the virus known as H5N1 and its potential to develop into a pandemic. Some in the scientific community are questioning whether that will ever happen.[1] If H5N1 does become pandemic, we have no basis for predicting whether it will be this year or 10 years from now. After all, H5N1 was first identified in birds in 1961; the first human cases did not appear until 1997.

There is little doubt, though, that eventually something—most likely a virus—will mutate into a pandemic form. The SARS outbreak in February 2003 is a good example of how a lethal virus can emerge suddenly. We were fortunate that SARS, while contagious, did not become pandemic.

The SARS outbreak and the emergence of H5N1 avian influenza provide us with a forewarning of the problems a larger outbreak will pose. It is prudent to use this time before the storm to plan for the societal disruption a pandemic will cause.

A pandemic poses problems that most disasters—even "ordinary" public health disasters—do not present. First, the time period of the disaster is extended; the 1918 pandemic lasted about 18 months, with three distinct peaks of infection and illness. Another issue with a pandemic is its geographic spread; modern air travel can deliver any pathogen worldwide in a very short time frame. Thus, our planning has to take into account the necessity to change our social behaviors and possibly restrict our movements to limit the pathogen's spread.

Preparing for the Storm

Limiting contact with our fellow humans for possibly a year and a half is a daunting task, but possibly necessary to save human life. However, in the midst of it all, society must continue to function. This document is a guide to help you prepare your organization for survival during a pandemic. All organizations have their own culture and character, so no one easy-to-follow guide will provide all of the answers for your specific group. This document is designed to provide you with resource materials from which you may pick and choose to tailor a plan that is best suited to your circumstances.

---

[1] Peter Palese, "Influenza Virus Pandemics: Past and Future," presentation at MIT Workshop on Pandemic Influenza: Science and Policy, June 15, 2006.

The significant findings and recommendations of this paper are provided in separate sections. A brief synopsis of each section is presented below.

Learning from the Past: The Pandemic of 1918

The pandemic of 1918 was the single most deadly outbreak of disease in the 20th century—possibly in human history. An estimated 500,000–675,000 Americans died; worldwide deaths were estimated at upwards of 50 million. The disruption to both society and commerce was virtually incalculable. The major lesson learned from the 1918 pandemic is the importance of planning to protect your organization's greatest asset—its people.

Making the Workplace Safe

From your organization's perspective, the pandemic will present a *readiness* issue—the availability of your workforce—*not* a medical issue. In order to ensure you have the maximum workforce available, the first priority is to make the workplace as safe as possible. Vaccines and anti-viral medications probably will not be available—at least not early in the pandemic—so classical, non-medical public health measures will offer the greatest security. To ensure a healthier workspace, we advocate the following:

- Emphasize basic personal hygiene practices, such as hand washing.
- Disinfect and sterilize work surfaces.
- Rearrange the workspace to place distance between people.
- Restrict or limit movement, activities, and gatherings.

Additional measures that will add to workplace safety preparedness include:

- Use of alcohol-based hand sanitizers (not to be confused with anti-bacterial soap).
- Ensuring an ample supply of tissues and disposal receptacles.
- Moving to a "paperless" society—avoiding circulation of unnecessary documents.
- Designating home and remote work locations (telecommuting).
- Inserting "infectious disease control" clauses in contracts—ensuring that those with whom you do business have tight controls to prevent the spread of disease (particularly important for businesses serving multiple buildings, such as contract cleaning crews).

Managing the Workforce

Managing the available workforce will pose tremendous challenges. Three sets of psychological responses can be expected. The primary response is fear. Obviously, everyone will have a level of anxiety and fear about contracting the disease. A secondary response will be discrimination against groups who may be perceived as spreading the disease. A tertiary response will manifest itself in those who suffer psychological trauma indirectly, by simply hearing or reading about flu-related incidents. At the group level, various "tipping points" may be reached, such as loss of faith in leaders and the belief that available assets are not being distributed fairly. These points may significantly influence group behavior. Identifying informal group leaders may help keep the workforce organized, and those leaders may serve as trusted sources of information. Establishing help lines and providing grief counselors are two other considerations for managers.

Communicating with the Workforce

There is *nothing* more important than the manner in which information is passed to the workforce. Succinctly, it involves four simple, but very sophisticated steps:

- Avoid errors in decisions and messages.
- Maintain trust in the sources of information.
- Avoid amplifying the risk.
- Encourage individuals, communities, and families to use coping mechanisms.

Keeping your workforce well informed will help reduce the level of anxiety and fear. Thus, the manner in which you handle risk communication is critical. Risk communication, however, is not just telling people the "facts;" it is also about the prospect of loss and about relationships.

Writing Your Plan

A pandemic is not a hurricane and an organization's "hurricane plan" cannot be adapted to fit the flu. Hurricanes and other similar natural disasters are usually characterized by being isolated in time and space, with extensive infrastructure damage. A flu pandemic, by definition, will be worldwide and will likely be longer lasting in duration than a natural disaster. The 1918 pandemic lasted 18 months, with three distinct peaks of increased morbidity and mortality. Thus, the response to a pandemic will be distinctly different from the response to a singular, catastrophic event. The Federal Government has issued its implementation plan for pandemic flu and calls for all sectors of society to prepare. Specifically:

- *Individuals Must Actively Participate.* Simple infection-control measures, including hand washing and staying home when ill, are critical. Individuals should actively participate in their communities' responses.
- *State and Local Governments Must Prepare.* Pandemics are global events, but individual communities experience pandemics as local events. State and local governments, with clear guidance from the Federal Government, should be prepared to implement community-wide measures, such as school closures and suspension of public gatherings, to halt the spread of disease.
- *The Private Sector Must Prepare.* The private sector, with targeted and timely guidance from the Federal Government, should develop plans to provide essential services even in the face of sustained and significant absenteeism. Businesses also should integrate their planning into their communities' planning.

After your organization's pandemic plan is written, it must be tested. Simple "tabletop" exercises are a good way to look for points of "friction." Several tabletop exercises may be necessary, using the employees who wrote the plan to role-play more senior officials. Once the plan is ready, a tabletop exercise that includes senior level players from your organization may be in order.

Additional Considerations

There are a multitude of additional considerations and each organization will have their own unique challenges. Some topics to consider include:

The Workload: Conduct an analysis of the tasks required for your organization to continue operating and prioritize them. Concentrate on ensuring that those tasks labeled as "mission essential" can be met, even if only half of your staff is available. Begin cross-training employees so that everyone is familiar with the mission-essential tasks and can perform them.

Proportionate Absenteeism: If your organization's work can be accomplished over the Internet, then office absenteeism does not necessarily mean eight hours of work will be lost each day an employee is absent. Some workers will be home sick and unavailable for work. Some workers will be well, but needed at home to care for those who are ill. Depending upon the circumstances—severity of illness and number of ill at home—an absent employee may be able to complete a few hours of work during a day. Some workers will be well, but unavailable due to fear or the need to care for children out of school. They may still be available for a full or partial day's work.

24-Hours a Day: If possible, establish a 24-hour work cycle. By moving to eight-hour shifts, the number of people at your workplace could be cut to one-third—significantly aiding the effort to establish social distancing.

Establish Help Lines: Identify phone lines and numbers that will be dedicated to employee help lines. Identify those individuals who will man the help lines and begin training them now. Have the help lines established at the lowest possible level—that is, each distinct group within your organization would have a specific number to call, and the group members would know the person answering the phone.

Review Personnel Policies: There may be legal or regulatory implications to your plan, and now is the time to discover that. In addition, your workforce will need to fully understand policies on leave and telecommuting.

The Golden Egg: An estimated $114 billion was spent preparing U.S. public and private sector computer networks for Y2K, and some estimate that worldwide Y2K expenditures may have exceeded $600 billion.[2] As companies began correcting their computer code

---

[2] U.S. Senate, Special Committee on the Year 2000 Technology Problem "Y2K Aftermath—Crisis Averted," February 9, 2000. Available online at <http://www.senate.gov/~bennett/issues/documents/y2kfinalreport.pdf>.

for the Y2K problem, they found other unnecessary code that could be eliminated, resulting in substantial savings in data storage and processing costs. Further research indicates that share value also improved as a result of the Y2K preparation.[3] Just as spending for Y2K resulted in unexpected benefits for corporate America, there may be an upside to preparation for pandemic flu—the chicken with bird flu may wind up laying a golden egg.

Preparing the workplace for telecommuting may mean large expenditures on information technology (IT) upgrades that will eventually result in increased productivity. High-speed Internet connection may have to be guaranteed for each employee's home, and web-based applications may need to be improved and used more broadly. A 2001 survey noted that almost three-fourths of managers polled reported slightly or greatly increased productivity from employees who worked at home. About one-fifth of managers felt that productivity stayed about the same, and only about six percent felt that it declined.[4]

Getting Started: A number of websites have been created that show plans for specific organizations. It is doubtful that any of these plans will be exactly right for your organization. However, plagiarism is not a crime in this instance! Take what looks applicable.

Tabletop Exercises: Putting your organization's plan to a test is a good way to find those points of "friction" that may cause it to fail when used in an actual situation. A number of websites have been developed with tabletop exercises that can be adapted to fit your organization's particular needs.

Enclosed at the back of this document is a CD that contains the following files:

- *Weathering the Storm*—an electronic version of this entire document.
- *Bird Flu and You*—an electronic version of the poster by the same name found on page 49.
- *Wall Poster*—a hyperlink to a website with details for obtaining a larger, more detailed flu poster.
- *Getting Started*—a collection of hyperlinks to COOP plans as listed in Appendix 1 of this document.
- *Tabletop Exercises*—a collection of hyperlinks to tabletop exercises as listed in Appendix 2 of this document.

---

[3] Krishman and R. Sriram, "An Examination of the Effect of IT Investments on Firm Value: The Case of Y2K-Compliance Costs," *Journal of Information Systems*, 2000, Fall, 95-108.
[4] "Is It Time to Dump Your Desktop?" *The Wall Street Journal*, July 24, 2006, R1.

Learning from the Past: The Pandemic of 1918

The 1918–1919 influenza pandemic was the single most deadly outbreak of disease in the 20th century, spreading in three distinct waves. The first wave of the virus occurred in the late winter and early spring of 1918, near the end of World War I, causing mild occurrences of influenza both in the United States and across the globe. The first wave was quickly followed by highly fatal second and third waves in the fall and winter of 1918–1919.

The first known instance of disease in the United States occurred in late January and early February 1918 in Haskell County, Kansas, where it is believed to have then spread to Camp Funston, the second largest army camp in the country. Housing an average of 56,000 troops preparing to deploy to Europe and other locations to fight in World War I, thousands of soldiers in Camp Funston became sick with influenza, resulting in 237 cases of pneumonia and 38 deaths.[5]

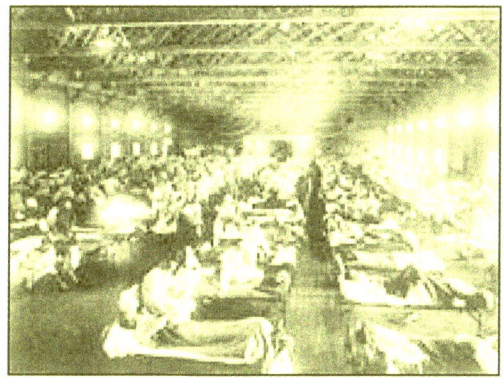

Emergency hospital during 1918 influenza pandemic, Camp Funston, Kansas.

From Haskell County, Kansas, it is believed that the virus spread to other military encampments in the United States and Europe with the deployment of American troops. The first unusual outbreaks of influenza in Europe occurred in Brest in early April 1918 with the arrival of American troops; nearly 40 percent of the two million American troops who arrived in France disembarked in Brest.[6] From Brest mild outbreaks of the virus began to appear in France, Germany, England, and Spain, spreading along routes of troop deployment, shipping lines, and trade routes.

Beginning in August 1918, near the end of the war, a highly virulent and lethal strain of the virus began to sweep the globe, appearing in India, China, Japan, and Southeast Asia, killing thousands. The illness was commonly, but incorrectly, referred to as "Spanish Flu." This name came from the fact that the earliest reports in Europe were reported in Spanish newspapers. Unlike other papers in Europe, which were heavily censored because of the war, the Spanish press was free to report on the illness and high death rates. Cases of influenza in the United States from this second wave of illness first appeared in Boston and Camp Devens, Massachusetts, in late August and early September.

[5] John M. Barry, *The Great Influenza: The Epic Story of the Deadliest Plague in History* (New York: Penguin Books, 2004), 96.
[6] Ibid, 182.

One of the catalysts for the spread of the deadly Spanish flu in the United States appears to have been from the Commonwealth Pier in Boston, MA, where the Navy operated barracks for sailors in transit. According to research conducted by John Barry, as many as 7,000 American soldiers ate and slept in the severely overcrowded quarters. Soldiers first began reporting sick at the Boston Commonwealth Pier on August 27, 1918.[7] The virus

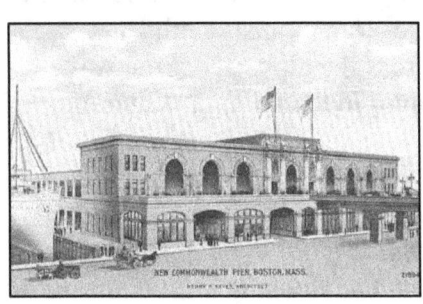

The New Commonwealth Pier in Boston, MA, was one of the catalysts for the spread of the deadly Spanish Flu in the United States.

then began to rapidly appear in other locations up and down the East Coast, including Camp Dix, New Jersey, and Camp Meade, Maryland. At Camp Grant outside Rockford, Illinois, the base hospital went from 610 occupied beds to over 4,100 in only six days and at Camp Custer, outside Battle Creek Michigan, 2,800 troops reported to the sick ward in a single day.[8]

The influenza virus continued to spread to military bases and cities throughout the United States with the movements of troops across the country, causing massive illness and thousands of deaths.

Relief and medical efforts to stop the spread of the disease in many cities were severely hampered due to a lack of supplies and a severe shortage of nurses and other volunteers healthy enough to care for those infected with the influenza virus. Hospitals were quickly overfilled with the sick and dying, and ill people lined up for hours in hopes of receiving medical care. Due to a shortage of healthcare personnel and available space in hospitals, however, thousands were turned away daily. During the epidemic, many cities, states, and counties enforced restrictions on public gatherings and travel to try to stay the epidemic. Churches and schools were closed, and one U.S. town even outlawed shaking hands. Other towns placed armed guards at the borders to keep outsiders from entering.

The second wave of the influenza pandemic peaked and began declining worldwide by the end of December 1918. Some countries, including the United States, experienced a third wave of disease in January and February 1919. Before the year was out, about 28 percent of the U.S. population had suffered from the Spanish Flu.[9] The estimated population of the United States on July 1, 1918 was roughly 103 million; approximately 0.5 percent of the U.S. population died as a result of the epidemic.

Usually the largest mortality from the seasonal flu comes in the very young and the very old. But in 1918, healthy men and women between the late teens and early thirties were the hardest hit. As shown in figure 1, the death rates for 15–34 year-olds dying of influenza and pneumonia were 20 times higher in 1918 than in previous years. The effect

---

[7] Ibid, 183.

[8] Carol Byerly, *Fever of War* (New York: NYU Press, 2005), 76.

[9] Carl Vinson Institute of Government, University of Georgia, "Chronology of the 1918 Spanish Influenza Epidemic in Georgia," April 7, 1999. Available online at <http://www.cviog.uga.edu/Projects/gainfo/1918flu htm>.

of the influenza epidemic was so severe that the average life span in the U.S. was depressed by 10 years.[10]

Figure 1: Influenza Mortality Curves

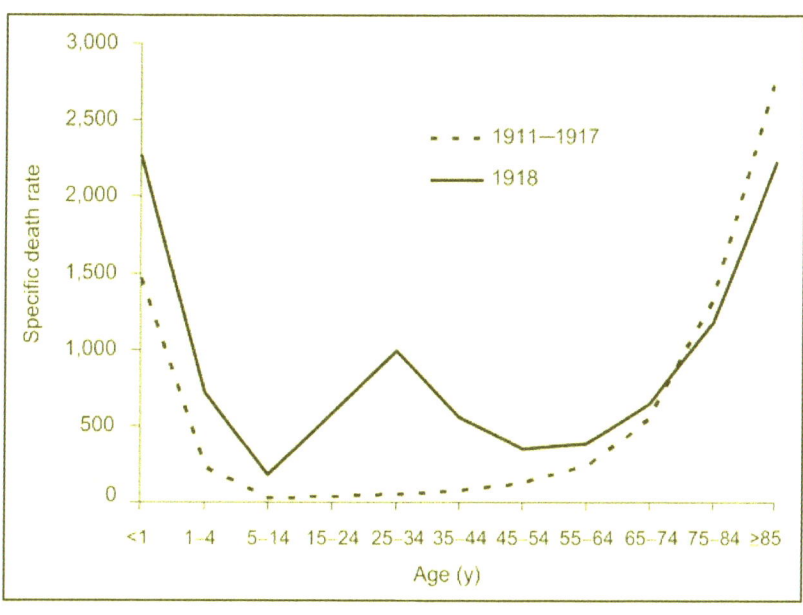

"U" and "W" shaped combined influenza and pneumonia mortality, by age at death, per 100,000 persons in each age group, United States, 1911–1918. Influenza-and pneumonia-specific death rates are plotted for the interpandemic years 1911–1917 (dashed line) and for the pandemic year 1918 (solid line).

Source: J.K. Taubenberger and D.M. Morens, "1918 Influenza: The Mother of All Pandemics." *Emerging Infectious Diseases*, vol 12, no 01, January 2006. Available online at <http://www.cdc.gov/ncidod/EID/vol12no01/05-0979.htm>.

By the end of the pandemic, an estimated 500,000–675,000 Americans had died and upwards of 50 million people had died worldwide. More people died of influenza in a single year than in four years of the Black Death (Bubonic plague) from 1347–1351.[11] The United States and the rest of the world had been exposed to such epidemics in the past, but never at such a severe cost in human life. Evidence indicates that the 1918 influenza pandemic was caused by an H1N1 avian influenza virus that was transmitted to humans. Since the 1918 influenza pandemic, two more influenza pandemics have occurred, in 1957–1958 and 1968–1969. While neither of these pandemics had as high a mortality rate as the 1918 influenza outbreak, they still caused significant loss of life.

---

[10] National Academies, Board on Global Health, "The Threat of Pandemic Influenza: Are We Ready?" Workshop Summary, 2005. Available online at
<http://www.nap.edu/openbook/0309095042/html/74.html>.
[11] Molly Billings, "The Influenza Pandemic of 1918," June 1997. Available online at
<http://www.stanford.edu/group/virus/uda/index html>.

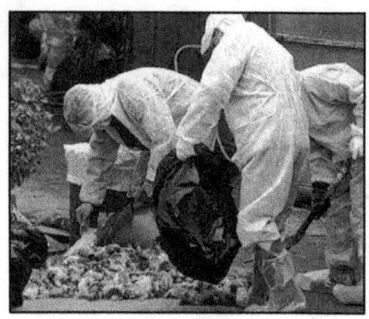
Officials cull chickens in Hong Kong markets in 1997 in an attempt to stop the spread of avian influenza.

The 1918 pandemic virus scenario presents a chilling comparison for recent H5N1 influenza outbreaks and virus transmission patterns in Asia. In 1996, a strain of avian influenza was first detected in geese in China's Guangdong province, and by 1997, a massive epidemic of avian influenza virus in poultry had broken out in Hong Kong. The first bird-to-human transmission of H5N1 occurred in Hong Kong during this outbreak, resulting in 18 infections and six deaths. In response to the outbreak, Hong Kong destroyed its entire poultry population of 1.5 million birds in three days. This is thought to have averted a pandemic by immediately removing opportunities for further human exposure.[12]

Since 1997, the H5N1 avian flu has continued to spread throughout Asia and into Europe, and by 2006 had appeared in birds in Austria, Egypt, Pakistan, and Romania, just to name a few of the latest countries that have been affected. Consequently, the pervasive threat of a pandemic outbreak in humans grows larger and more imminent.[13] This is further compounded by the fact that many countries lack infectious disease surveillance capabilities and modern health systems.

Improved influenza surveillance in influenza "hot spots" needs to be instituted. Along with increasing disease surveillance capacity, replacing economic disincentives to early reporting of disease with incentives for surveillance, and timely disease detection, access to vaccines and antiviral drugs will greatly increase the chances of recognizing and containing an emerging pandemic strain before or soon after it emerges.[14]

The financial implications of the 1918 pandemic are difficult to fully estimate, as available economic data are limited, at best. The pandemic occurred during WWI, when most governments restricted the flow of information. Additionally, economic data are limited for the time period because national income accounting was in its infancy.[15] Even absent firm data, it is safe to say that the economic losses to businesses were felt throughout the world. Merchants suffered because customers were too ill to shop, staff were absent with the flu, and transportation was halted. Pool halls, restaurants, and theaters all lost heavily.[16] According to available data, both industrial production and the business activity index in the United States dipped in October 1918, at the height of the pandemic.

---

[12] R. Webster and D. Hulse, "Controlling Avian Flu at the Source," *Nature*, 2005, 435:415-6.
[13] S.M. Lemon and A.A.F. Mahmoud, "The Threat of Pandemic Influenza: Are We Ready?" *Biosecurity and Bioterrorism: Biodefense Strategy, Practice and Science*, 2005, 3:70-3.
[14] Ibid.
[15] International Monetary Fund, "The Global Economic and Financial Impact of an Avian Flu Pandemic and the Role of the IMF," February 28, 2005. Available online at <http://www.imf.org/external/pubs/ft/afp/2006/eng/022806.pdf>.
[16] K. Duncan, *Hunting the 1918 Flu: One Scientist's Search for a Killer Virus* (Toronto, Canada: University of Toronto Press, 2003).

Not surprisingly, evidence shows that consumption in the United States fell during the pandemic. As a result, the proportion of the population that contributed to savings increased. In the decade following the pandemic, the rate of economic growth increased approximately two percent per year. Some feel that because incomes fell during the pandemic years, the observed economic growth that followed was attributable to a return to pre-pandemic economic growth patterns.[17]

Based on the disease patterns of post-World War II pandemics, a new flu pandemic could cause 100,000–200,000 deaths in the United States, together with 700,000 or more hospitalizations, up to 40 million outpatient visits, and 50 million additional illnesses. Scholars at the World Bank have stated that the present value of the economic losses associated with this level of death and sickness is estimated at between $100–$200 billion for the United States (in 2004 dollars), with the potential worldwide economic cost of a pandemic topping U.S.$800 billion over the course of a year.18 Others estimate the worldwide economic costs of an avian flu pandemic could reach U.S. $4.4 trillion—a global gross domestic product (GDP) decline of 12 percent.[19]

While many lessons can be learned from the 1918 pandemic, the issue of human capital stands out. Aside from the human element related to the suffering, the notion that so many people in the workforce could be absent at one time raises serious questions about continuity of operations (COOP). Unlike many other catastrophic events, an influenza pandemic will not directly affect the physical infrastructure of an organization. A pandemic will not damage power lines, banks, or computer networks; however, it will ultimately threaten all of society's institutions by its impact on an organization's human resources. Essential personnel could be removed from the workplace for weeks or months. Employers should include considerations for protecting the health and safety of employees during a pandemic in their business continuity planning. Because the movement of essential personnel, goods, and services and the maintenance of critical infrastructure are necessary during an event that spans weeks to months in any given community, effective continuity planning is a "good business practice" that must become part of the fundamental mission of all plans.[20]

---

[17] E. Brainerd and M. Siegler, "The Economic Effects of the 1918 Influenza Epidemic," September 2002, Available online at
<http://scholar.google.com/scholar?hl=en&lr=&q=cache:HwmohhX9HZkJ:faculty.econ nwu.edu/faculty/fe rrie/wksp/Sept%252026th.pdf+1918+influenza+economic+loss>.
[18] M. Brahmbhatt, "Avian and Human Pandemic Influenza—Economic and Social Impacts," November 2005. Available online at
<http://web.worldbank.org/WBSITE/EXTERNAL/NEWS/0,contentMDK:20715087~pagePK:34370~piPK :42770~theSitePK:4607,00.html>; World Health Organization, "Avian Flu: Economic Losses Could Top US$800 Billion," November 8, 2005. Available online at
<http://web.worldbank.org/WBSITE/EXTERNAL/COUNTRIES/EASTASIAPACIFICEXT/EXTEAPREG TOPHEANUT/0,,contentMDK:20715408~menuPK:503054~pagePK:34004173~piPK:34003707~theSiteP K:503048,00 html>.
[19] The Economist, "Big Questions and Big Numbers," July 15, 2006, 67.
[20] White House, "The National Strategy for Pandemic Influenza- Implementation Plan," May 2006. Available online at <http://www.whitehouse.gov/homeland/nspi_implementation_chap09.pdf>.

Influenza Naming Convention

There are three types of influenza: A, B, and C. Influenza A viruses (which include the avian viruses) cause the most severe disease in humans. Influenza B can infect humans and seals. Although it can be lethal and cause epidemics, it is not known to cause pandemics. Influenza C viruses are not known to cause epidemics and only cause mild disease.

Influenza A viruses are further identified by sub-type, based on the types of proteins that are on the virus' surface. The hemagglutinin protein (H) aids the virus in gaining entry into a cell. There are 16 possible variants of hemagglutinin. The neuraminidase protein (N) helps new virus particles escape from a cell, once it has multiplied. There are nine possible variants of neuraminidase. All of the possible combinations of H and N subtypes (e.g., H1N1 (cause of the 1918 pandemic), H5N1, H7N7, etc.) can infect birds. With respect to the H subtypes, humans have only been known to be infected by H1, H2, and H3. Thus, the H5N1 virus is new for humans.

Making the Workplace Safe

From an organizational perspective, a flu pandemic will not be a medical issue, but rather a readiness issue. That is, normal staffing levels will be affected. Some estimates suggest that as many as 40 percent of a workforce may not be present.

For those who are present, it is imperative to make the workplace a safe and comfortable environment. It is unlikely that direct medical actions, such as providing vaccinations or antiviral medications, will be adequate or sufficient enough to fully protect your workforce. It is unlikely that public health officials will have all that much to offer in the form of medicines, at least in the early stages of a pandemic. Thus, non-medical steps will provide the most effective measures to control the spread of the virus and provide a secure workplace.

Why Medicine Will Not Provide the Total Response

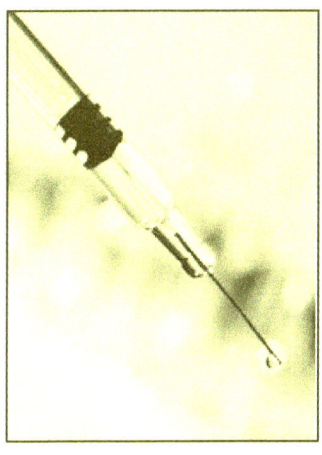

Large-scale production of an effective vaccine is unlikely early in a pandemic.

Faced with the threat of H5N1 (the agent currently identified as causing avian flu or bird flu) as a precursor for a human pandemic, there has been, and will continue to be, considerable focus on medical responses to the threat. This focus has included both vaccinations and the use of antiviral agents for both prophylaxis and treatment. Prophylaxis is defined as "preventative medicine or course of action," but can be readily thought of as the pre-treatment use of appropriate drugs. In the case of H5N1, this will comprise vaccine and antiviral products. For an H5N1-derived pandemic influenza episode, consideration of prophylaxis using antiviral drugs is a contentious issue, in part because of the limited stockpiles of the drugs.

Vaccines are considered the first line of defense in reducing illness and death during an influenza pandemic. More than ten countries around the world have domestic vaccine manufacturers, many of which are working on the development of a pandemic influenza vaccine.[21] Unfortunately, the large-scale production of a vaccine effective against a flu pandemic is unlikely to be available until at least six months after a pandemic has started. By that time, the first and perhaps also the second wave of a worldwide pandemic likely would have occurred.

The United States Government has awarded a number of contracts for vaccine production and some candidates have shown promise during clinical trials. To date, however, no vaccine has been manufactured that is considered to be the final answer to the problem.

---

[21] World Health Organization, "Vaccine Research and Development: Current Status," November 2005. Available online at <http://www.who.int/csr/disease/avian_influenza/vaccineresearch2005_11_3/en/index html>.

Research is also underway to include adjuvants in a vaccine. Adjuvants are substances that boost the immune response. Theoretically, limited supplies of vaccine could go further if they were adjusted to provide the lowest effective dose, which an adjuvant would make possible.

Another factor to consider is that the current H5N1 virus is *not* causing a pandemic. In order to do so, it will need to undergo genetic change. Commercial production of a vaccine cannot begin prior to the emergence and identification of the structure of the virus in a pandemic form. The actual vaccine will need to be a close match to the pandemic virus.

Four antiviral medications that could potentially be used for the treatment and prophylaxis of pandemic influenza are commercially available in the United States. The drugs are classified into two categories: neuraminidase inhibitors (oseltamivir and zanamivir) and adamantanes (amantadine and rimantadine).[22] The neuraminidase inhibitors, zanamivir (Relenza) and oseltamivir (Tamiflu) appear to be effective against currently circulating strains of the H5N1 virus; however, they have a limited production capacity and may be too expensive for many countries to afford.

The second class of drugs, adamantanes, have not been effective against the current H5N1 virus strains circulating in Asia and Europe. These strains have developed antiviral resistance to both the adamantine drugs amantadine and rimantadine. This raises concern over the future development of antiviral resistance to other drugs, including the neuraminidase inhibitors. Research is currently underway to develop novel antivirals that could treat avian influenza.

With only limited medical supplies, there is understandable concern in some quarters about whether sufficient amounts of these resources will be available during an outbreak—especially if the outbreak occurs in the near future, when the resources are extremely scarce. There has also been concern about how effective medical countermeasures may be against the H5N1 virus, given the ability of this virus to mutate, and its proven capability to become resistant to antiviral drugs.

Non-Medical Interventions

Against this backdrop, interest is growing in implementing non-medical interventions that would include:

- Basic personal hygiene practices.
- Disinfection and sterilization of surfaces.
- Social distancing (SD).
- Movement and activity restrictions (MAR).

---

[22] World Health Organization, "Antiviral Drugs: Their Role during a Pandemic," November 2005. Available online at <http://www.who.int/csr/disease/avian_influenza/antivirals2005_11_3/en/index.html>; Anthony S. Fauci, "Pandemic Influenza Threat and Preparedness," *Emerging Infectious Diseases*, vol. 12, no. 1, January 2006.

These well-established public health measures have a long history of successful use against a range of human diseases. They are also the mainstay of the public health measures that were used to "control" the outbreaks of SARS in countries around the world. Measures such as basic hygiene practices and disinfection or sterilization are often described as basic common sense. Their inclusion in any planning for responses to a pandemic episode would appear to be straightforward. But only through explicit inclusion in the communications with the members of your organization will these measures be widely adopted. Your organization's members, as well as the general public, will need to be reassured that, as basic as they appear, non-medical interventions represent concrete actions that can reduce transmission of the virus. If used appropriately, they will save lives. Simple they may be, but simple, effective measures will be invaluable against H5N1.

Although many of these non-medical interventions were tested during the emergency response to SARS, their use during the different conditions of an influenza pandemic has not been systematically evaluated. Consideration of their use during a pandemic is particularly important, as non-medical interventions will be the principal protective tools so long as supplies of effective vaccines and antivirals remain scarce. In countries unable to secure adequate supplies, non-medical measures may be the main line of defense throughout the course of a pandemic.

In a 2004 report, the World Health Organization (WHO) noted that the effectiveness of many interventions will depend on the behavior of the virus as determined by its pathogenicity, principal mode of transmission (droplet, aerosol, or contact), attack rate in different age groups, duration of virus shedding, and susceptibility to antivirals.[23] If, for example, it is known that children are the most severely affected age group, or play a major role in transmission, health authorities will be in a better position to make decisions about the effectiveness of school closure, travel measures (children travel less frequently than adults), and quarantine (children cannot be separated from their parents). Apart from questions of effectiveness, the selection of appropriate measures will be driven by questions of feasibility closely linked to costs, available resources, ease of implementation within existing infrastructures, the broader impact of possible interventions, and likely acceptability to the public.

WHO examined the full spectrum of public health responses and their application in a pandemic disease event. The report noted that, when faced with a pandemic situation, the general public would probably be strongly motivated to adopt personal protective measures and behaviors, some of which may have limited effectiveness. It was felt that these measures should be permitted, provided they caused no harm and did not have major resource implications.[24]

In reviewing past outbreaks of highly infectious diseases, including the pandemic influenza of 1918, the public health utility of SD and MAR is of little doubt, but

---

[23] World Health Organization, "Avian Influenza: Assessing the Pandemic Threat," January 2005. Available online at <http://www.who.int/csr/disease/influenza/WHO_CDS_2005_29/en/>.
[24] Ibid.

scientific, social, and cultural issues surround the implementation of some of these measures in any society. This is particularly the case in the United States where the rights of citizens to individual and collective freedoms and liberty are enshrined in the Constitution and all facets of everyday life. In developing recommendations, it will be important to evaluate the likely protective effect of specific measures and consider the resource implications and the social and economic disruption they might cause.

Notwithstanding the concerns noted, it is likely that multiple forms of SD and MAR will be used in the event of a pandemic influenza public health emergency, and that such use will have psychological and psychosocial impacts on the affected individuals and their communities.

It also will be important to consider compliance with recommended (or even enforced) public health measures. During a time of pandemic flu, several key categories of behaviors will greatly impact the spread of disease and the ability of the public health and health care system to provide care to those affected. All of these behaviors fall on a continuum such that one's behavioral reaction to the emergent disease threat could be considered desired or undesired; for example, washing one's hands is a desired behavior while failing to wash one's hands is an undesired behavior. Finding ways to promote adherence to public health recommendations will be vitally important in combating the disease.

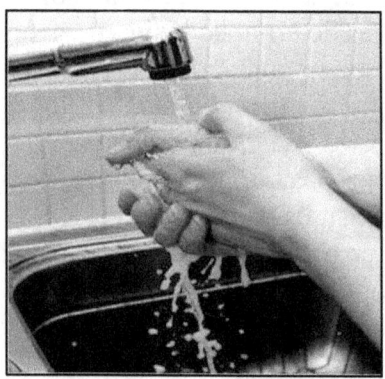

Hand washing is a simple, but effective way to control the spread of the flu.

Officials will also be concerned that those who present with influenza symptoms seek proper care at the appropriate time and that those without symptoms, particularly individuals who make up the critical workforce infrastructure (e.g., medical personnel, teachers, and first responders), continue their daily routine as directed. During a period of pandemic influenza, the public health community will stress the importance of universal hygiene and wellness behavior, including hand washing, cough etiquette, receiving adequate sleep, exercising, and eating a balanced diet.

Hand washing, in particular, is one of the most important actions that can protect against illness and prevent the spread of infection in an influenza outbreak (pandemic or seasonal). Compliance with this simple instruction will be another matter entirely. In a survey of hand washing behavior sponsored by the American Society for Microbiology, although 95 percent of adults claim that they always wash their hands after using public restrooms, only 78 percent were observed doing so.[25] Among youth, the percentage is even smaller. In one study, only 58 percent of female and 48 percent of male middle and high school students washed their hands after using the bathroom, and, of these, only 28 percent of the females

---

[25] Wirthlin Worldwide, "A Survey of Hand Washing Behavior," American Society for Microbiology, September 2003. Available online at <http://www.washup.org/survey.html>.

and 8 percent of the males used soap.[26] It would seem that even simple behaviors can be difficult to promote with a skeptical or overburdened population.

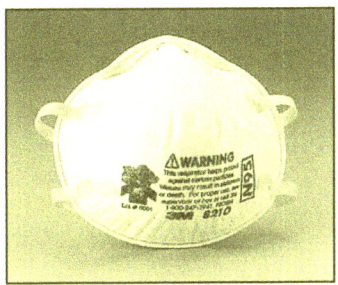

While debate will continue about whether masks are effective for everyday use during an H5N1 pandemic, it is clear that wearing a mask will not cause harm (N-95 mask pictured).

Equally, debate can be considerable about the merits, or lack thereof, of even "simple" public health measures, including the use of masks during a pandemic outbreak. In the opinion of WHO experts, the use of personal protective equipment may reduce but not eliminate the possibility of being infected with H5N1. However, experts not only continue to debate about the utility of masks for everyday use, but also the effectiveness of surgical and N-95 masks—the type worn by construction workers—during a pandemic influenza outbreak. In part this is driven by a concern that no scientific or medical evidence proves that masks are effective against the H5N1 virus. This evidence-based standard could be considered too rigid, given that complete data to support a decision on masks will not be documented until after an H5N1 episode.

Current data suggest that the virus would be transmitted between humans by three major routes:

- Droplet (respiratory secretions) transmission, which is common among close (within one meter) contacts. (E.g., an infected person sneezes or coughs and the secretions enter the mouth, nose, or eyes of a susceptible person.)
- Aerosol transmission, where virus-containing particles are inhaled by a susceptible person.
- Contact (respiratory secretions) transmission, which may occur through hand-to-mouth or hand-to-eye transmission after touching an influenza virus-contaminated object or surface.

Masks will significantly reduce droplet (and possibly aerosol) transmission and could, thus, be considered valuable as a public health control mechanism. (At least one researcher suggests that masks could even help control contact transmission by keeping hands away from mouth and nose.)[27] While debate will continue about whether masks are effective for everyday use during an H5N1 pandemic, it is clear that wearing a mask will not cause harm.

With regard to the third method of transmission (contact with infected surfaces), disinfection and sterilization are both proven to be effective. The difference between disinfection and sterilization is that disinfecting a surface removes or kills some, but not

---

[26] M.E. Guinan, M. McGuckin-Guinan, and A. Sevareid, "Who Washes Hands after Using the Bathroom?" *American Journal of Infection Control*, 1997; 24(5): 424-425.

[27] L. Wein, "Face Facts," *The New York Times*, October 25, 2006. Wein further states that his research suggests the dominant mode of transmission will be aerosol, thus possibly reducing the value of hand washing.

all disease causing microorganisms, whereas sterilizing a surface kills every microorganism. The H5N1 influenza virus is inactivated by alcohol and chlorine. Cleaning of environmental surfaces with a neutral detergent (e.g., laundry detergent, hand soap) followed by a disinfectant solution (e.g., bleach, alcohol) is recommended.

In summary, the physical setting of your workplace can be organized to help limit the spread of H5N1, simply by practicing a few commonsense measures. Consider the following:

- Reorganizing the workspace to give greater distance between workers.
- Providing alcohol-based hand sanitizer dispensers (*not* to be confused with antibacterial soaps, which may actually make the workforce more susceptible to certain bacterial infections).
- Keeping work surfaces clean.[28]
- Providing ample supplies of tissues and appropriate disposal receptacles.
- Moving to a "paperless" environment by sending materials electronically to limit the amount of paper passed around.
- If possible, encourage telecommuting. Now is the time to establish secure websites for your organization.

The potential "Typhoid Mary" that could create a pandemic is the employment of contract security, cleaning, and other facility service providers and suppliers. Many organizations hire, for example, crews that clean multiple buildings during the course of a day. While managers and employees may take extraordinary precautionary measures against the transmission of H5N1 influenza, the cleaning crew or other contract workers might be the vector that carries contamination from another worksite.

During the Y2K preparation, a standard clause began appearing in many contracts, requiring companies to certify that their computer systems were "Y2K compliant." Thus, if your company had spent considerable time and money preparing for Y2K, your efforts would not be undermined because of an affiliation with the computer network of another company that was not prepared.

In a similar vein, organizations should begin inserting "infectious disease control" clauses in contracts. Such clauses would guarantee that sound public health measures were being taken by those companies with which they did business. While it would be no guarantee that contamination would be completely avoided, it would provide an economic incentive for companies to ensure their practices were sound. Such clauses should not be limited to cleaning crews, as all partners are potential sources of contamination.

---

[28] Influenza A and B viruses have been shown to survive on hard, nonporous surfaces—stainless steel and plastic—for one to two days. On cloth, paper, and tissues, they were shown to survive for at most 12 hours. Measurable quantities of influenza A virus were transferred from stainless steel surfaces to hands for 24 hours and from tissues to hands for up to 15 minutes. Viruses survived on hands for up to five minutes after transfer from environmental surfaces. (J. Bean, et al., Infectious Disease, 1982 Jul; 146(1):47-51.)

The Chicken Who Laid the Golden Egg...Maybe

Remember January 1, 2000? It is not especially memorable because of what did *not* happen. Civilization as we know it did not come to an end. Despite all of the dire warnings about Y2K and the "millennium bug," most computers rolled over and treated it like the day it was. That was no accident, however. An estimated $114 billion was spent preparing our public and private sector computer networks for the big day. Some estimate that worldwide expenditures for Y2K preparation may have exceeded $600 billion.

Was all that expenditure really necessary? After all, as was pointed out at the time, although everyone knew what the risks were, nobody was completely certain as to what the ultimate impact would be. However, as companies began correcting their computer code for the Y2K problem, they found other unnecessary code that could be eliminated—resulting in substantial savings in data storage and processing costs. Not only did it result in cost savings for firms, it also added to the overall value of the companies. Krishnan and Sriram, two researchers, note: "We find that estimates of Y2K-compliance costs were positively and significantly related to share prices...the stock market is not shortsighted, and considers investments in Y2K-remediation efforts a significant and value-increasing activity for the average firm."

Just as spending for Y2K resulted in unexpected and positive benefits for corporate America, preparation for pandemic flu may have an upside. Preparing the workplace for telecommuting may mean large expenditures on IT upgrades. For example, high speed Internet connection may have to be guaranteed for each employee's home. The Government Accountability Office (GAO) reported in May 2006 that currently only 28 percent of American households have broadband service. In addition, web-based applications may need to be improved and used more broadly. The current suite of web-based products that compete with the larger packages generally available on desktops are not fully acceptable to all businesses—especially larger ones. In addition, laptops may need to be purchased for employees.

Once a company has prepared its workforce for telecommuting, however, the potential for increased productivity is considerable. A 2001 survey from the International Telework Association and Council noted that almost three-fourths of managers polled reported slightly or greatly increased productivity from their employees who were working at home. About one-fifth of managers felt that productivity stayed about the same, and only about six percent felt that productivity declined. The impetus for spending money to remove old code was preparation for Y2K. Similarly, the impetus for preparing the workforce for telecommuting may be pandemic preparedness. In the end, the chicken with bird flu may eventually be the source of a golden egg for your organization, as the pandemic expenditures may well prove as beneficial to organizational efficiency as the Y2K expenses.

Sources: U.S. Senate, Special Committee on the Year 2000 Technology Problem "Y2K Aftermath— Crisis Averted," February 9, 2000. Available online at <http://www.senate.gov/~bennett/issues/documents/y2kfinalreport.pdf>; Richgard Bergeon, "Y2K: Leadership in an Emergent Crisis." Available online at: <http://www.ila-net.org/Publications/Proceedings/2003/rbergeon.pdf>; G. V. Krishnan and R. Sriram, "An Examination of the Effect of IT Investments on Firm Value: The Case of Y2K-Compliance Costs." *Journal of Information Systems*, 2000, (Fall), 95-108; GAO, "Broadband Deployment is Extensive Throughout the United States, but It Is Difficult to Assess the Extent of Deployment Gaps in Rural Areas," GAO-06-426, May 2006; "Is It Time to Dump Your Desktop?" *The Wall Street Journal*, 24 July 2006, R1; Smart Commute @RTP, "Productivity Graph of Telecommuters." Available online at <http://www.smartcommute.org/TelecommutePL.htm>.

Managing the Workforce: Epidemic Psychology

Introduction

Configuring the workplace during a pandemic will be an easy issue in comparison to managing the workforce. Employees will be under stress for a variety of reasons. Many may be dealing with sick family members or even grieving the loss of loved ones. Moreover, people may be asked periodically to restrict their movements, further causing stress in their daily lives. Additionally, many may find themselves, willingly or not, placed in a situation at work where they have to help someone who has become critically ill. Your workforce members may also find themselves "pressed into service" to assist in a variety of duties to support public servants. Understanding these problems will help in keeping the workforce healthy, both physically and mentally.

Public health measures used to manage a disease outbreak often include wide-ranging and mandatory interventions and stringent prohibitions on the day-to-day activities of people affected by, or potentially affected by, an emergent disease. Examples of mandatory public health interventions used in past outbreaks include: quarantines, vaccination or treatment, physical examination or diagnostic testing, travel restrictions, and epidemiological investigations, among others.

These interventions can impact rights and freedoms that people consider protected under the U.S. Constitution and that they consider inviolable. The measures can also generate areas or issues of considerable tension between the public and their appointed officials and have in the past been the focus of public unrest during disease outbreaks.

Based on the range of interventions that could be invoked during a pandemic episode, it is very likely that social disruption and possibly violence will be a major concern. Against this background of increased public unrest we are faced with the fact that personnel who could be used for enforcement of the public health measures will have to be drawn from a wider pool than just local and state law enforcement officials, as many of these likely will be suffering from influenza. With limited local and state capabilities on hand for deployment to areas of concern, National Guard forces, if available, are anticipated to play a key role in augmenting law enforcement personnel. This may serve to increase the tension between a scared public and those seeking to restore order and structure to the public health response.

Under these circumstances, any actions that will minimize the negative reactions of the public and generate behaviors that are beneficial to the impacted communities will be of great value. In this section the issues that would exacerbate the incident and contribute to negative responses are explored; measures that could potentially elicit positive social behaviors are also discussed.

In a 2004 exercise that examined the impact of a disease on a population (in this case the impact of smallpox), the situation was eloquently explained by a former U.S. senator. "The Federal Government has to have the cooperation from the American people. There

14

is no Federal force out there that can require 300 million people to take steps they don't want to take."[29] Why do we need to consider the psychological and psychosocial responses? Because we need cooperation from the public. If we fail to understand the emotional response to the outbreak, our actions will not be targeted at cooperation and we will not succeed.

Many of the issues and strategies described here are common sense, but by making them explicit and incorporating them into the plans, policies, and procedures that are being considered for a pandemic episode, they become powerful tools for program planning and evaluation of mechanisms to mitigate the impact of a pandemic influenza outbreak.

The analysis of the public response to a pandemic can be usefully divided into psychological and psychosocial domains. In the context of this paper this distinction attempts to characterize the two domains as relating to individuals and their mental health state (psychological) and those of the larger society (psychosocial). While such divisions may appear arbitrary, they are tightly linked and interdependent. In a later section of the paper consideration is given to the conflict that exists between individual and community centric action. The ability to generate positive psychological responses that in turn drive beneficial psychosocial behaviors is a valuable asset. The fact that improved societal conditions will help with individual psychological reactions is also discussed. Clearly, any response to the outbreak will benefit from understanding the responses of individuals and communities.

Likely Psychological Impacts

The experiences with SARS would appear to be valuable when evaluating the likely impact of an H5N1 outbreak. Considerable data have been published on the immediate and currently discernable psychological impacts of SARS. There is also evidence that the psychological and psychosocial impacts were qualitatively and quantitatively affected by the geographic location in which the disease occurred.

A pandemic influenza episode resulting from the rapid human-to-human transmission of the H5N1 virus will generate significant psychological and psychosocial reactions in the general population. Chief among these reactions will be a fear of being unwittingly infected by a diseased individual. Other significant features that will generate concern are the fact that the disease could be fatal, that there will be limited antiviral drug treatments and vaccines, and that the public health management of the disease will include significant restrictions on day-to-day activities of individuals and some larger segments of the population.

Aside from the direct experience of the outbreak, which in the case of a pandemic will be extensive, very few people will be unaffected. Most people will have family connection to areas where the disease is occurring, thus raising the level of psychological reaction to

---

[29] Former Senator Sam Nunn, playing the U.S. President in *Dark Winter*, the June 2001 smallpox bioterrorist exercise, *Biosecurity & Bioterrorism*, 2(1):25-40, 2004.

15

the outbreak. In fact, one of the unique features of a pandemic influenza episode is the geography of the incident. Most incidents or disasters (whether naturally-occurring or man-made) have distinct foci where the major impact is located. A pandemic episode will not be so constrained and will affect large parts of the country as well as around the globe at the same time. Under these circumstances the public will be participants in the incident rather than spectators of the event. Firsthand experiences of a pandemic will be widespread, almost universal. This represents a unique challenge to incident managers, responders, and the victims. The absence of a defined, and all too local, focus for the incident will present significant psychological and psychosocial challenges to the public and those responsible for the response.

For populations that have become used to seeing public health response in terms of antibiotics and vaccines, the pictures shown in figure 2 convey a response to the disease that is much more frightening. Images of facemasks, isolation suits, and disinfectant crews, accompanied by commentary suggesting enormous uncertainty about the disease in terms of its effects, lethality, and mode of spread, raised significant questions in populations hearing about SARS for the first time. Similar reactions can be anticipated for any future pandemic influenza episode.

Figure 2: Images from the SARS Outbreak

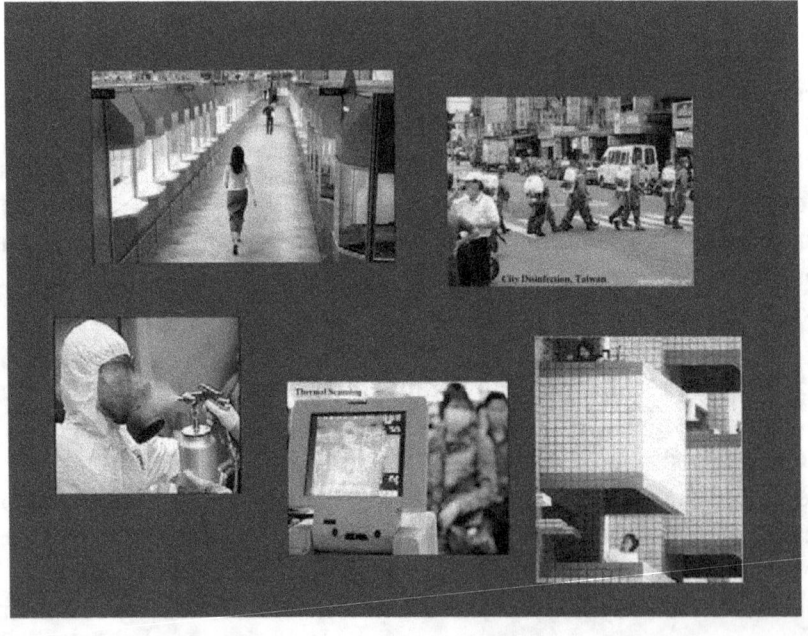

Lessons can be learned from the SARS outbreak to help inform our planning for a pandemic influenza. The images that were broadcast by media outlets around the world provided a stimulus for the psychosocial response to the disease, which should be taken into account when planning for a pandemic influenza event.

Recent research from Canada relating to the SARS outbreak documents that even within a specific location, the specifics of the public health response, the availability of information, and the socioeconomic status of the affected persons all had an effect on the extent and degree of the psychological after effects.[30] It is important to note that factors including geographical location, culture, local and state governments, legal statutes, and economic status will shape public health responses and public behavioral patterns. The differences between states within the United States represent significant factors that will need to be considered when Federal resources are used to provide public health management of the outbreak. These differences may prove to be significant in terms of how a public, faced with a pandemic influenza episode, may respond to the imposition of public health measures that could impact their lives in several adverse ways.

For the purposes of reviewing the psychological and psychosocial impacts that would result from a pandemic outbreak, three areas of response provide key elements for analysis.

Primary Responses: Any disease state has a range of key criteria that influence the psychological reactions of the public. Many diseases evoke reactions characterized by fear or dread of disease. Regardless of the risk to an individual or his or her immediate family, these basic concerns can lead to changes in behavior and psychological reactions that can complicate the public health management of the disease state.

Secondary Responses: Many diseases that are initially identified in discrete communities, but that have an ability to spread beyond that community, elicit psychological reactions that are characterized by stigmatization, discrimination, and other concerns that can manifest in antisocial behavior and further complicate the public health management of the disease state.

Tertiary Responses: The disease can adversely impact not only individuals who are directly affected, but also those who are made aware of the disease through direct knowledge of an infected person or by hearing or reading about the disease from media sources or the Internet. The immediate psychological and psychosocial impacts in this case are influenced by many factors but may be amplified if the disease also evokes either of the primary or secondary responses described above. The tertiary responses can also be influenced by the requirements for medical or public health responses to address the specific concerns of the disease state. The implementation of either, or both, a medical or a public health response may evoke individual, community, or even national concerns that can have psychological and psychosocial impacts that transcend the disease state and may have long-term implications.

It is worth noting that if the disease has evoked, or can invoke, strong primary or secondary responses, the tertiary responses can be significantly magnified and can lead to pronounced psychological and psychosocial impacts. The latter manifestations may be so strong that they can even lead to psychosomatic manifestation of the disease symptoms in

---

[30] L. Hawryluck, W.L. Gold, S. Robinson, S. Pogorski, S. Galea, and R. Styra, "SARS Control and Psychological Effects of Quarantine," *Emerging Infectious Diseases*, 2004, vol. 10 (7).

individuals who have had no direct exposure to the disease and across large portions of the general population. In the case of some diseases, particularly where the onset is rapid and mediated by a specific event or through rapid person-to-person infection, the public response can be a significant concern and represent an additional medical management component that can absorb considerable resources and require specific actions to mitigate. Psychosomatic responses create their own reality and attendant problems—not the least of which is misuse of vital, and often scarce, resources.

The relationship between the three types of response is shown in figure 3, which indicates that, over time, the psychological responses, composed of the primary, secondary, and tertiary elements, increases. The psychosocial component of that response begins with reactions to the initial description of the disease, continues with response to the identification of the affected persons, and culminates in the response to the management of the disease through implementation of public health measures. The magnitude of the psychological response is determined by the individual primary, secondary, and tertiary responses. Moreover, the period of time in which the component responses are manifest will be different for each disease and the population it impacts. For example, the annual epidemic of influenza in the United States typically exhibits a horizontal-type model of response—the fear of the disease (primary response) causes only a mild response. With influenza the public reaction includes "we have seen this before," and "we've had our flu shots." Neither reaction by the affected population normally provokes a strong secondary response. Finally, the public health response to influenza is usually characterized by public health announcements that limit the tertiary response.

Contrast the *normal* response with that of the 2003–2004 influenza season, when it was announced in the media that the virus had a propensity to cause fatalities in children. The response model for influenza shifted to a more *vertical* model—the magnitude of the psychological response and the timeframe were very different from the norm. An influenza that was *different* increased the magnitude of the primary response, the belief that the virus affected children magnified the secondary response, and the shortage of vaccine led to an increased tertiary response. We now have a model of increased psychological response over a shortened timeframe and are beginning to shift from a controlled reaction by the public to one showing early signs of a panic.

Figure 3: Modeling the Psychosocial Impact

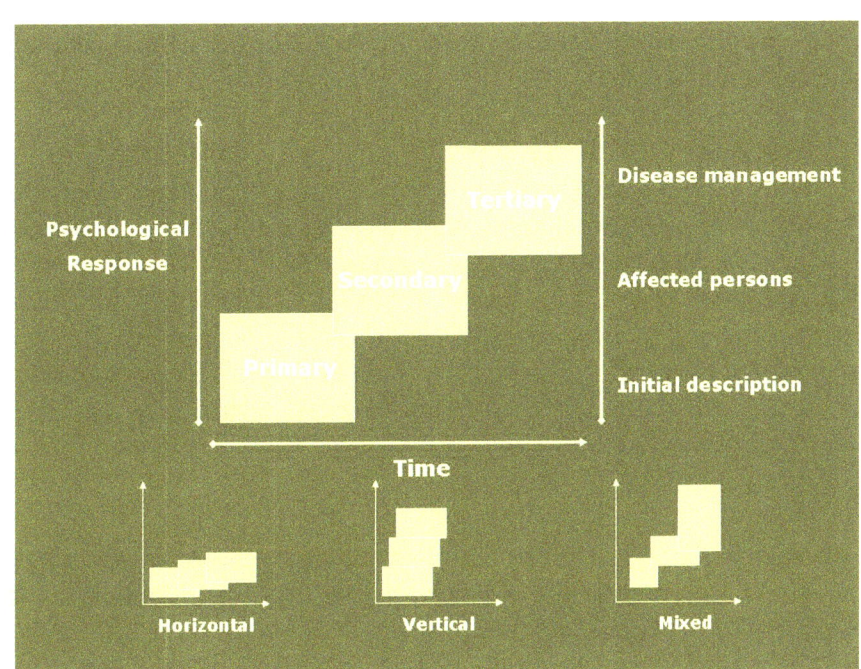

Model of increased psychological response over a shortened timeframe.

Understanding how the model can affect both the scale of the psychological or psychosocial responses and how that can impact the extent and composition of the required resources to manage the situation are important elements in developing an effective plan for responding to any incident that is generated by a disease state.

Primary Responses: Fear and Dread of Disease—Epidemic Psychology

The experiences with SARS dramatically illustrate the first area of concern when considering the likely psychological and psychosocial impact of a new pandemic episode.[31] In the article "Fear and Stigma: The Epidemic Within the SARS Outbreak," the authors noted that, "Fear of SARS arose from the underlying anxiety about a disease with an unknown cause and possible fatal outcome." They also noted that, "Fear is further fueled when infection control techniques and restrictive practices such as quarantine and isolation are employed to protect the public's health."[32]

The SARS outbreak exhibited much less severe psychological and psychosocial impacts than a future pandemic influenza will. Nonetheless, it demonstrated a pronounced psychological and psychosocial impact because of two factors that will also be present in

---

[31] B. Person, F. Sy, K. Holton, B. Govert, and A. Liang, and the NCID/SARS Community Outreach Team, "Fear and Stigma: The Epidemic Within the SARS Outbreak," *Emerging Infectious Diseases,* 2004, vol.10 (2).
[32] Ibid.

any future pandemic episode. The first of these is the rapid and widespread transmission of information about the outbreak, especially information about causality, such as how the disease is spread. The second component is the lack of medical information about treatments and infection control.

Phillip Strong wrote one of the most compelling descriptions of fear and dread of disease in a review that first used the term "epidemic psychology."[33] In his review, Strong argued that the early reaction to major fatal epidemics constitutes a distinctive psychosocial form, which he named epidemic psychology. He also noted that its underlying micro-sociology may well be common to all such diseases but is manifested in its purest shape when a disease is new, unexpected, or particularly devastating. Strong also suggested that his model of epidemic psychology is directly rooted in some fundamental properties of human society and social action. He gave as his principal example the response to AIDS, but the model readily translates to the SARS outbreak as well as any possible future episode of pandemic influenza.

Epidemic psychology is a phrase with a double meaning. It contains within it a reference, not just to the special micro-sociology or social psychology of epidemics, but to the fact that psychology has its own epidemic nature, quite separate from the epidemic of disease. Like a disease, it too can spread rapidly from person to person, thereby creating a major collective as well as individual impact. At the same time, its spread can take a much wider variety of forms. Epidemic psychology, indeed, seems to involve at least three types of psychosocial epidemic.[34]

The epidemic of fear seems to have several striking characteristics, or potential characteristics. First, the epidemic of fear is also an epidemic of suspicion. There is the fear that *I* might catch the disease and the suspicion that *you* may already have it and might pass it on to me. A second characteristic of novel, fatal epidemic disease, seems to be a widespread fear that the disease may be transmitted through any number of different routes, from sneezing and breathing, to dirt and other day-to-day items. A third striking feature, closely linked to the two above, is the way that fear and suspicion may be wholly separate from the reality of the disease.[35] One striking feature of the early days of such epidemics seems to be an exceptionally volatile intellectual state. People may be unable to decide whether a new disease or outbreak is trivial or really something important.

Strong concludes that epidemic psychology can only be conquered when new routines and assumptions that deal directly with the epidemic are firmly in place, a process that requires collective as well as individual action. Thus, any pandemic influenza plan must seek to address the primary psychological and psychosocial responses that may be evoked by providing authoritative data about the disease and its medical and public health management before the next occurrence. It will not be sufficient to respond to the

---

[33] Philip Strong, "Epidemic Psychology: A Model," *Sociology of Health & Illness*, 1990, vol. 12 no. 3.

[34] The first of these is an epidemic of fear. The second is an epidemic of explanation and moralization and the third is an epidemic of action or proposed action.

[35] Classically associated with this epidemic of irrationality, fear, and suspicion is an epidemic of stigmatization.

initial reports of a new outbreak of the disease because with the speed of today's information flow the public will already be developing ideas, actions, and responses that may negatively impact the management of the outbreak.

Secondary Responses: Stigmatization and Discrimination

In general, it has been observed that following the recognition that a disease has the ability to impact individuals or communities, those with the disease, and those who belong to what are feared to be the main carrier groups, can both be stigmatized. This can begin with avoidance, segregation and abuse, and progress to significant levels that may even lead to acts of violence against persons or property. All kinds of disparate but corrosive effects may occur. Friends, family, and neighbors may be feared, with strangers being feared above all the other groups. The sick may be left uncared for and those believed, even if incorrectly, to be carriers of the virus may be shunned or persecuted. Moreover, it is worth noting that such avoidance, segregation, and persecution can be quite separate from actions aimed at containing the epidemic.

In a very well researched article, Nelkin and Gilman note that:[36]

> Despite the sophisticated scientific understanding underlying concepts of disease in the late twentieth century, we still seek explanations based on behavior, ethnicity, or social stereotypes. We still use disease to protect our social boundaries or to maintain our political ideals. And, at a time when control over disease is limited, we still blame others as a way to protect ourselves. By drawing firm boundaries, that is, by placing blame on "other groups" or on "deviant behavior," we try to avoid the randomness of disease and dying, to escape from our inherent sense of vulnerability, to exorcise the morality inherent in the human condition.

In a recent publication, the authors noted that, "Studies have shown that during serious disease outbreaks, when the general public requires immediate information, a subgroup of the population that is at potentially greater risk of experiencing fear, stigmatization, and discrimination will need special attention from public health professionals."[37] The SARS outbreak was a classic example of such an outbreak. During the SARS outbreak, for example, some individuals became fearful or suspicious of all people who looked Asian, regardless of their nationality or actual risk factors for SARS, and expected them to be quarantined. Fear of being socially marginalized and stigmatized as a result of a disease outbreak may cause people to deny early clinical symptoms and contribute to their failure to seek timely medical care. It has also been noted that stigmatization associated with discrimination often has social and economic ramifications that intensify internalized stigmatization and feelings of fear.

---

[36] Dorothy Nelkin and Sander Gilman, "Placing Blame for Devastating Disease," *Social Research*, 1988, vol. 55, no. 3.
[37] B. Person, et al.

Unlike the SARS outbreak, the wide geographical spread of a pandemic disease state will encompass most of the world's population. There will not be a focus on specific populations who can be identified as being "responsible" for the spread of disease or who represent a higher risk from infection. This will diminish the stigmatization and discrimination component of the psychological and psychosocial responses to the incident. However, it is worth noting that some professions and activities will engender a closer association with infected persons. The people engaged in these activities may be perceived as representing a higher risk of transmitting the disease and result in them being targets of stigmatizing or discriminatory actions by other people.

It is important to note that during the 2003 SARS outbreak one of the groups that was identified as experiencing significant episodes of stigmatization and discrimination were healthcare workers and their families. The fact that these people were risking their lives to try and treat disease sufferers did not make them immune from the base reactions of persons who did not want to have direct contact with persons who may be able to transmit the disease. The incidence of SARS in healthcare workers was initially higher than anticipated, however, a shift in the medical practices for handling and contacting infected patients was an effective control strategy and reduced the rates in the latter stages of the outbreak. Nonetheless, the impact of the disease on such a critical resource was significant and added to the burden of the medical management of the outbreak. In plans for future incidents, the possibility that healthcare workers and other firstline responders may become victims of the secondary responses to the disease state need to be built into the communication and education plans for informing not only the general public, but also these critically important assets in our fight against the disease.

Tertiary Responses: Disease and Disease Management Impacts

The tertiary psychological and psychosocial responses of individuals and communities result from two factors: the impact of the disease and the perception of the impact of the medical and public health responses to the disease.

In the latter case the word perception is used advisedly—the actual impact that imposed measures will have on any individual or group may not be as important as the perceived impact. Many of the responses that have occurred were not born out of the reality of their effects but by the perception of their possible impact. As noted previously, fear of the unknown plays a role in the public's reaction to the disease state and the intervention measures.

The Individual versus Citizen Conflict

In a 2003 article Baruch Fischhoff wrote that:

> Terrorism has created unprecedented choices for ordinary people. As individuals, they must decide how to protect themselves and their families. As citizens, they must decide which policies best serve the nation's desire for physical safety, economic vitality, civil liberties, and social cohesion. Without good information, people may find themselves living with choices that they do not understand or want. Feeling that they have been denied critical information further complicates an already difficult situation. If things go badly, having misunderstood the risks can intensify the attendant pain and regret.[38]

The same dichotomy will exist for individuals who are subject to the imposition of public health responses to pandemic influenza. This is one of the key issues that will drive the psychosocial impact of the response to the disease state. The problem of resolving the conflicts inherent in this issue are much more personal than those normally raised when consideration is made of the potential impact of disease management measures like quarantine. For the most part the issues of the "common good" are set against the issue of "civil liberties"—these are important and critical issues, but for the average person the fundamental issue will be the conflicts in personal choice as shown in figure 4.

Figure 4: Conflicts in Personal Choice

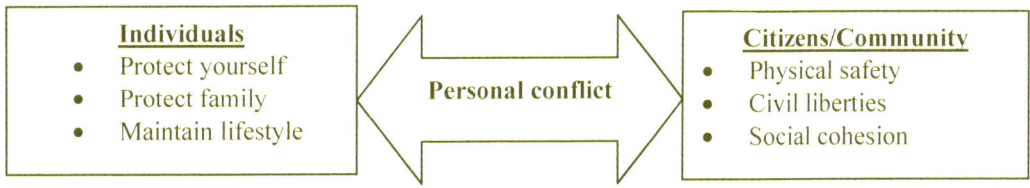

The average person will be faced with conflicts by having to balance what is good for him or her on an individual level versus what is needed for the "common good."

Any plan to help mitigate or manage the psychosocial issues presented by a response to a disease that includes movement restrictions must address this issue and others that relate to it.

It is also important to note that one component of the response to other bioterrorism or public health threats, which will not have a significant role for pandemic influenza, is the deployment of the strategic national stockpile (SNS) of medical products. The limited resources in the SNS to combat H5N1 influenza will likely cause confusion in some

---

[38] B. Fischhoff, et al, "Evaluating the Success of Terror Risk Communications," *Biosecurity & Bioterrorism*, 2003, vol. 1 (4): 255.

portions of the population and may even result in increased anxiety based on the perception that "not everything is being done to help us."

Counter-productive psychological and behavioral health responses to a disease outbreak can impede response efforts. During an influenza pandemic, for example, both psychological and psychosomatic distress responses (e.g., grief, anger, fear, depression, and psychosomatic illness) and behavioral changes may decrease an individual's ability to adopt and adhere to public health measures that minimize personal exposure and/or disrupt disease transmission in the community. In addition to the potential health consequences, maladaptive emotional and behavioral responses can create disruptive and disastrous economic results, overtax the health care system, and incite stigma and discrimination.

Reported Psychological and Behavioral Consequences Following Incidents such as Terrorism and Disease Outbreaks

- ❖ Psychological Distress.
- ❖ Fear and Suspicion.
- ❖ Psychiatric illness.
- ❖ Multiple Unexplained Physical Symptoms (Psychosomatic Illness).
- ❖ Stigmatization and Discrimination.
- ❖ Altered Behavior and Perceptions.
  - o The use of tobacco, alcohol, and drugs.
  - o Perceptions about danger and safety.
  - o Routine activities.
  - o Civic or faith-based organizational involvement.

Source: D. B. Reissman, E. A. Whitney, T. H. Taylor, Jr. et al. "One-year health assessment of adult survivors of Bacillus anthracis infection," *JAMA, 2004,* 291: 1994-1998.

The historical accounts of the 1918 pandemic flu abound with descriptions of a disease that exhibits frightening characteristics. These will undoubtedly create psychological and psychosocial reactions that will hamper the public health management of the outbreak and severely disrupt the day-to-day lives of the population.

Additional characteristics of pandemic influenza that must be considered when assessing potential psychological and behavioral health impacts include:

- Simultaneous impacts in communities across the United States, thereby limiting the ability of any jurisdiction to provide support and assistance to other areas. Communities face the possibility of responding to influenza with minimal external resources or support—or none at all.[39]

---

[39] Ibid.

24

- An overwhelming burden of ill persons requiring hospitalization or outpatient medical care.
- Likely shortages and delays in the availability of vaccines and antiviral drugs.
- Disruption of national and community infrastructures including transportation, commerce, utilities, and public safety.
- Global spread of infection with outbreaks throughout the world. With the world's growing, and increasingly urban-based population, the speed and volume of travel provides a basis for widespread and rapid transmission of disease.
- Responses between affected countries will differ significantly. Some will rapidly respond to a shift in the disease state while others will be more reticent and their inaction may precipitate a much bigger problem.[40]

There is also concern that in the United States the public perception of influenza as "an annual inconvenience that causes transient sickness in young adults with limited mortality in the very young and very old" is inconsistent with the possible characteristics of a pandemic influenza. This disconnect will be further exacerbated by the expectation on the part of the public that an influenza outbreak should be readily managed by the advanced and modern health care system in operation in the United States. If the pandemic targets the critical population of young adults in the health care arena and is not adequately controlled by the healthcare system, the impact on the public may be profound.

Experiences with SARS confirm the potential significant impact that epidemic psychology will have on the general public, as well as first responders, incident managers, and the country's leadership. These experiences suggest that even a moderate pandemic episode will overwhelm current health care service capacity. The absence or severe limitation of such services will exacerbate the negative reactions from the public. To effectively manage the outbreak and decrease the psychological damage that results from a pandemic, the "managers" of any incident must seek to institute measures that:

- Maximize public trust and effectiveness of communication.
- Maximize adaptive behavior change.
- Reduce social and emotional deterioration and improve adherence and pro-social functioning.
- Maximize professional performance and personal resilience for key personnel in critical infrastructure.

---

[40] This was the case in the 2003 outbreak of SARS. The response from some countries was to suppress the fact that the disease had been detected. The resultant delay in response created an even greater problem in those countries, their neighbors, and around the world where the disease was spreading.

Tipping Points

According to author Malcolm Gladwell, a "tipping point" is "the boiling point." It is the moment on the graph when the line starts to shoot straight upwards.[41] In considering the psychological and behavioral health responses that could occur during pandemic influenza the tipping point concept becomes a very useful tool. In the context of the work described in this document we define a "tipping point" as: events, actions, or perceptions that strongly influence psychological reactions or social behaviors at the group level.

It is important to note that the definition encompasses, either positively or negatively, both the reality and the perception of the events or actions. Distinguishing between reality and perceived reality may be valuable before or after an incident, but at the time the episode is occurring, those people most at risk will be directly aware of only their own situation and that of their family and community. All other "realities" will be viewed through one or more filters of the media-based and non-media coverage of the episode. In the latter category a multitude of information sources (official, unofficial, regulated, unregulated, unintended rumors, and malicious rumors) will provide key stimuli for both positive and negative psychological and behavioral health responses.

Some important tipping points in a pandemic influenza are shown in the following box:

Psychological and Psychosocial "Tipping Points"

❖ Lack of information.
❖ Belief that resources are not available, fairly distributed, or effective.
❖ Ineffective or insufficient triage.
❖ Blame, stigma, and discrimination.
❖ Restriction of civil liberties, especially if restriction is perceived to be inequitable.
❖ Rumors and conspiracy theories.
❖ Loss of faith in social institutions and leaders.
  o Especially medical, public health and social systems of care.
  o Includes law enforcement and life safety.
❖ Economic hardship driven by outbreak management procedures.
❖ Excessive impact on self, family, or children.

The recognition of specific tipping points that would influence a disease outbreak in the United States is an important component in managing counter-productive psychological and behavioral health responses and is a major focus in the work described below.

---

[41] Malcolm Gladwell, *The Tipping Point: How Little Things Can Make a Big Difference* (Boston: Little, Brown and Company, 2000).

After assessing the likely tipping points, measures that would counter the negative actions and accentuate the positive actions brought on by the tipping points can be identified, as well metrics to assess whether the countermeasures were succeeding or failing. The suggested countermeasures are summarized in the following box.

Psychosocial and Behavioral Countermeasures—Focus Areas

❖ Measures to shape adaptive behaviors.
  ○ Guidance about maximizing public trust and effectiveness of communication.
  ○ Guidance to maximize adaptive behavior change.
❖ Measures to reduce social and emotional deterioration and improve functioning.
  ○ Public information, guidance, and support aimed at increasing hope, safety, connectedness, and personal/community efficacy.
❖ Measures to support key personnel in critical infrastructure functions (e.g., healthcare, emergency responders, child-serving, utilities, food).
  ○ Maximizing performance and resilience (managing grief, exhaustion, anger, fear, family and self-care issues, and resolving ethical dilemmas).

Group Leadership

Obviously, group leadership is going to be key to maintaining a physically and mentally healthy workforce in the midst of a pandemic. Of all the definitions of leadership, perhaps the most succinct and appropriate one to this situation is that given by Stratford Sherman: leadership is the ability of a person to influence human behavior in an environment of uncertainty.[42] The formal leaders may not be the ones who help your organization weather the storm of a pandemic. Formal leaders are selected for their skills in helping the organization achieve its goals. However, those same skills may not be applicable to meeting the psychological needs and demands of your workforce during a pandemic. The necessary leadership skills may come from unexpected, informal leaders.

Informal leaders who arise to maintain employee mental health will likely be those who are compassionate, good at listening, empathetic, good at communicating, and able to place people ahead of the mission. While these are worthy skills for anyone in a formal leadership position, they may not be ranked as highly as the analytical abilities or strategic thinking skills usually prized in senior management. Thus, an informal leader, or group of leaders, may arise within the organization to help meet the special psychological needs likely to result from a pandemic.

---

[42] Stratford Sherman, "How Tomorrow's Leaders are Learning Their Stuff," *Fortune*, 1995, 132, (11), 90–102.

Identifying and training these informal leaders now is an important step. Many academic papers have been written on methods to identify informal leaders. For this particular need, however, use of peer interviews is probably the most efficient; using sources within the group is the best method of identifying who the true informal leaders are.[43] Informal leaders could be trained in how to deal with the psychological aspects of a pandemic and receive additional training so that they become trusted sources of technical information on the virus and methods of control. In addition to informal leaders, an organization might also consider placing a grief counselor on retainer. Such an addition could add significantly to your organization's ability to survive the emotional drain of a pandemic.

---

[43] Donald W. Knox, "The Importance of Informal Leaders in Organizations," 2005, Center for Collaborative Organizations." Available online at <http://www.workteams.unt.edu/literature/paper-dknoxjr.html>.

Telling It Like It Is: Communicating With the Workforce

Perhaps no area of preparedness is more important than the manner in which organizational leaders communicate with their workforce. Rumors and misinformation will abound in a pandemic. Credible, reliable and accurate information will be the key to controlling the spread of false ideas and help prevent "pandemic panic." Numerous sources of information will be available, and your organization has to carefully select its source(s). Also, spokespersons—those who speak to the workforce as well as those who speak to the public on behalf of your organization—must be carefully selected and trained.

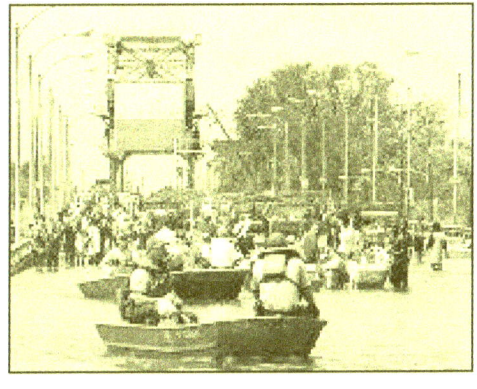

The experience of Hurricane Katrina demonstrates the necessity for effective communication.

The potential for an influenza pandemic poses new challenges for communicating risks. The experience of Hurricane Katrina in New Orleans demonstrates how a natural disaster can be compounded by media attention to human error (delays in responding), technical failure (levee breaks), and systems dysfunction (particularly in intergovernmental relations and the chain of command). These problems were amplified by round-the-clock news coverage in the aftermath of Hurricane Katrina.

This section is designed to look at communications challenges, a field where much has been learned from dealing with environmental and public health controversies over the past three decades. Effective communication is important in coping with crises involving infectious disease outbreaks. Undoubtedly, timely and accurate communication will be critical to ensuring public cooperation and understanding during a pandemic. Better communication has been viewed as a way to deal with such things as fear, frustration, helplessness, outrage, anxiety, and distrust.[44]

---

[44] V.T. Covello and P.M. Sandman, "Risk Communication: Evolution and Evolution," in A. Wolbarst, (ed) *Solutions to an Environment in Peril* (Baltimore, MD: Johns Hopkins University Press, 2001), 164-178; P. M. Sandman, "Hazard Versus Outrage in the Public Perception of Risk," in V.T. Covello, D. B. McCallum, and M.T. Pavlova, (eds) *Effective Risk Communication: The Role and Responsibility of Government and Nongovernment Organizations* (New York: Plenum Press, 1989), 45-49.

There are four key ways to improve risk communication:

- Agencies must avoid errors in decisions and messages.
- Officials must maintain public trust in sources of information.
- News organizations need to avoid amplification of risk.
- Officials must encourage individuals, communities, and families to use coping mechanisms, particularly protective steps.

For more than 30 years risk communication has evolved from a scientific focus (quantifying the probabilities of hazards) to one that increasingly looks to the cultural and social factors that influence risk perception. The National Academy of Sciences stated in 1989 that risk communication is "an interactive process" involving "multiple messages," including some "not strictly about risk," including "opinions" and reactions to legal issues and institutional management. The Academy's recommended approach is to treat people as partners in a dialogue with the leadership of interested groups to ascertain their concerns, fears, ideas, and demands and to agree on ways to address these issues.

Over the years of dealing with environmental health controversies it was realized that quantification of risk takes a backseat to quality of life and other value issues during such crises. Baruch Fischhoff has traced the evolution of environmental risk communication, listing some of the steps that official experts have tried over the years:[45]

- All we have to do is get the numbers right.
- All we have to do is tell them the numbers.
- All we have to do is explain what we mean.
- All we have to do is show them they have accepted similar risks before.
- All we have to do is show them it is a good deal for them.
- All we have to do is treat them nice.
- All we have to do is make them partners.

In his conclusion, Fischhoff states that all of the above need to happen before people will accept advice on how to cope with a new risk. If society does not communicate the dangers of both man-made and natural health risks, it is likely that there will be nothing "nice" about the way things like quarantines are imposed or evacuation is attempted in a future episode. It is here that the New Orleans hurricane experience is relevant: lessons can be learned from the way people were transported or forced into shelters without adequate provisions. In the case of a pandemic, it is not difficult to imagine that people trapped in inner cities and told they cannot leave their homes might feel abandoned and discriminated against.

Allegations of racism and unfair treatment of the poor surfaced in New Orleans due to mishandling of a flood; imagine a national health crisis where dozens of cities attempt to

---

[45] B.Fischhoff, "Risk Perception and Communication Unplugged: Twenty Years of Process," Paper for Addressing agencies' risk communication needs: a symposium to discuss next steps (Annapolis, MD: 1994).

restrict the movement of people. Risk communication efforts can be greatly compromised if the news media focus attention on the plight of unhappy victims. Unfortunately, most officials communicate in a way that ignores Fischhoff's last point about treating the public as "partners." Authorities tend to want to do the talking, rather than engage in dialogue with a scientifically uninformed public.

There are three ways to define communication: what *I* say, what *they* hear, and what *we* learn. Many people never get past the I-oriented view of communication to consider the impact of their messages on the audience. While the decision on what to say is very important, the focus should be on what the audience hears, remembers, and acts upon. Beyond that, communication is a two-way street and an important way that individuals— and society—learn. Therefore, communication must be considered a plural process. There are several purposes for communicating, including to inform, educate, persuade, motivate, manipulate, and coerce.

When people are first told of risks they often want unambiguous answers to the question: Is it safe for me and my family? Educating the public about scientific risk analysis is not what the public wants. Rather, it wants to know what should be *done* about the risk.[46] Clear and definitive answers are rarely possible. Dealing with uncertainty is difficult but essential. Since fear of the unknown increases the fearsomeness of risk, how can an official spokesperson address the unknowns without scaring the public unnecessarily? There is sometimes a temptation to keep people in the dark about small risks. However, if an organization hides information, it risks ruining its credibility when the problem is highlighted. If people suspect a cover-up, credibility can be destroyed and subsequent efforts at public communication will be hampered.

As environmental health problems became more complex and controversial, new insights were learned and skills taught to managers who had to face the public. Most of these controversies involved Government agencies such as the Federal Environmental Protection Agency (EPA), the Food and Drug Administration (FDA), the Occupational Safety and Health Administration (OSHA), and their counterparts in state and local governments. The overwhelming body of research into risk communication has centered on the risks caused by humans, with most of it being tied to specific technologies or risk events like accidents or unintended side effects of drugs or medical devices. More attention was paid to man-made risks than to diseases of a natural origin until the AIDS epidemic spurred efforts to prevent the spread of that disease. Nevertheless, public health agencies were largely spared the most bruising lessons about risk controversies that their counterparts in environmental agencies were experiencing. The threat of a pandemic or bioterrorist attack makes it important for public health specialists to understand how risk communication has evolved over several decades of environmental activism.

The agencies tasked with safety regulation differentiate between risk assessment, risk management, and risk communication. Risk assessment includes four steps: identification of a specific hazard, assessment of the relation between magnitude of exposure and the

---

[46] D. Powell and W. Leiss, *Mad Cows and Mother's Milk: The Perils of Poor Risk Communication* (Montreal, Canada: McGill-Queen's University Press, 1997).

probability of occurrence of a health effect, determination of the extent of human exposure under regulatory controls, and characterization of the nature and magnitude of human risk, including aspects of uncertainty.[47] In general, risk assessment attempts to quantify the actual risk. The next step in the process is risk management, which attempts to evaluate those risks against broader social and economic values. The National Research Council (NRC) stated in 1983, "At least some of the controversy surrounding regulatory actions has resulted from a blurring of the distinction between risk assessment policy and risk management policy."[48]

The NRC recommended that scientific findings and policy judgments in risk assessments should be explicitly distinguished from the political, economic, and technical considerations that influence the choice of regulatory policy. It is in risk management that the costs and benefits of policy choices are usually weighed. Risk communication was initially thought to be the final part of the process, when the public would be informed of the results of the assessment and risk management processes. Nothing so linear has ever worked. Usually decisions get driven by decibel level. An EPA Science Advisory Board stated in 1990 that "since public concerns tend to drive national legislation, federal environmental laws are more reflective of public perceptions of risk than of scientific understanding of risk."[49]

Here are some of the problems inherent in communicating with the general public about risks to health:

- Scientific studies are complex, jargon-laden, and filled with uncertainty. They rarely answer the layperson's question, "Is it safe?"
- Scientists and government officials are not in agreement about how to characterize risk, compare risks, rank risks, and prioritize regulatory action.
- Many risks are unprovable and policy preferences and assumptions influence the results in risk assessments.[50]
- Risk information is often communicated by advocates in activist groups, industry spokespersons, trial lawyers, and politicians who are perceived to have their own agendas and lack credibility with the public.[51]
- Businesses with products under attack often respond with defensive public relations, ranging from the inept to the deceitful.[52]
- Risk information becomes ammunition in the policy debate, in court battles and in the media.

---

[47] National Research Council, *Risk Assessment in the Federal Government: Managing the Process* (Washington, DC: National Academy Press, 1983).
[48] Ibid., 3.
[49] U.S. EPA, "Reducing Risk: Setting Priorities and Strategies for Environmental Protection," Report of the Science Advisory Board, September, 1990, 12.
[50] U.S. Department of Energy, "Choice in Risk Assessment: The Role of Science Policy in the Environmental Risk Management Process" (Washington, DC: Regulatory Impact Analysis Project, 1994).
[51] D. L. Burk, "When Scientists Act like Lawyers: The Problem of Adversary Science," *Jurimetrics Journal of Law, Science and Technology*, 1993, 33: 363-376.
[52] F. Rowan, "The High Stakes of Risk Communication," *Preventive Medicine*, 1996, 25: 26-29.

- The news media are interested in conflict and sensationalistic stories and errors often appear in news accounts.[53] Controversies about risk are easy to start and hard to resolve.[54]
- The general public has a high level of scientific illiteracy. Most people have read and watched more science fiction than have read and learned about science.
- The public often feels powerless, fearful and outraged upon hearing of a newly disclosed threat to public health and/or the environment. People want to protect themselves, so feelings of powerlessness are particularly problematic. Risk communication is about *values*, things that people care about. It is not just about technical measurement of hazards and their probabilities of harm. Psychological, social, and cultural explanations have been offered as competing theories to explain risk perception, but Kasperson and collaborators say that risk events interact with all three of these factors in ways that heighten or attenuate public perception and related risk behavior.[55]

Risk communication is also about the prospect of *loss*. People tend to be willing to expend more energy to avoid a loss of something they possess than they would expend to gain a new, equal amount of the same thing.[56] All things being equal, people fight to keep what they have with more vigor than they display when they are seeking something new. When cost/benefit analysis is performed by disinterested outsiders they might ask "What's the fuss?" But for someone who faces the loss of security, of neighborhood tranquility, and of his sense that his or her children are safe, that potential loss is felt so acutely that it can outrage people and motivate them to protect themselves.

Risk communication is about *relationships*. On one level it is about how people interact with technology, including hazardous substances and pharmaceuticals. On a deeper level it is about how people interact with other people—including the ones who treat the sick, manage the technologies, or regulate them. In a pandemic it will be about how people interact with their neighbors (who may be contagious) and emergency responders and health care providers. It is about people with a stake in the outcome of the discussion. Stakeholder interaction and competing values are at the heart of the controversies about risk.[57] Because the issues are laden with values—differing values—even in the best of times communicating about risk is a challenge.

Because risk communication is about values, potential losses, and relationships, it almost always is about *conflict*. Even at its most juvenile level, when children are told they must take their medicine, wash their hands, look both ways before crossing the street, or not

[53] E. Singer and P.M. Endreny, *Reporting on Risk: How the Mass Media Portray Accidents, Diseases, Disasters and Other Hazards* (New York: Sage, 1993).
[54] K.R. Foster, D.E. Bernstein, and P.W. Huber (eds), *Phantom Risk: Scientific Inference and The Law* (Cambridge, MA: MIT Press, 1994).
[55] R.E. Kasperson, O. Renn, P. Slovic, H.S. Brown, J. Emel, R. Goble, J.X. Kasperson, and S. Ratick, "The Social Amplification Of Risk: A Conceptual Framework," *Risk Analysis*, 1988, 8(2): 177-87.
[56] D. Kahneman and A.Tversky, "Choices, Values and Frames," *American Psychologist*, 1984, 39: 341–350.
[57] D. Von Winterfeldt and W. Edwards, *Understanding Public Disputes About Risky Technologies* (New York: Social Science Research Council, 1984).

touch the hot stove, there is room for resistance and it is expected. Grown-up scientists and policy-makers are rarely in agreement on how to characterize risk, compare risks, rank risks, and prioritize governmental actions. If conflict is such a challenge in the absence of an emergency, imagine the difficulty of communicating about risks of mass death.

For many people, complex health information is difficult to comprehend in a time of stress. One way people process risk information has been described by Sandman.[58] People tend to view risks in the context of their ability to control them. Voluntary risks are perceived as less risky than coerced risks. Risks that an individual has direct control over are deemed less risky than uncontrolled ones. Risks that are familiar seem less risky than unfamiliar ones. Risks that are judged to be "fair" are perceived as less risky than unfair ones. Additionally, risks that provide direct benefit seem less risky than ones with no payoff. These factors—familiarity, controllability, voluntariness, fairness, benefit— are about who knows, who decides, who pays, and who gets what; in short, about *power*. Put in a different way, things seem very risky when people feel powerless. An important part of risk perception involves people feeling left in the dark, deprived of choice, coerced into accepting uncontrolled risks, getting the short end of the stick. These feelings of political impotence are what drives outrage and leads people to reject the advice of experts and their technocratic assessments. What many people want is not to be told by officials what the scientific risks are, but to force the system to listen to and respond to their concerns.

Despite suggestions that the United States is becoming a more risk-averse society, there is little evidence to suggest that people will always demand zero risk. What people seem to fear the most—exotic chemicals, invisible radiation, new viruses—may pose a lower risk than the things people do the most—drive, smoke, drink alcohol—that kill hundreds of thousands of persons each year.[59] In fact, regulation must balance two opposing forces: the demand for protection and the demand for freedom of choice, including access to new technologies and products that offer some benefit.

One of the keys to successful risk communication is to empower people to choose the best alternative to reduce risk to themselves and their families. This requires a closer examination of the communication process. There are four aspects: issues regarding what is in the messages; the capabilities and credibility of the sources of information; the performance of the channel of communication, usually the mass media; and the comprehension of receivers of information, the general public. The following review builds upon this four-fold division of the problematic nature of risk communication.

---

[58] P. M. Sandman, "Definitions Of Risk: Managing The Outrage Not Just The Hazard," in T. A. Burke, N. L. Tran, J. S. Roemer and C. J. Henry (eds), *Regulating Risk: The Science And Politics Of Risk* (Washington, DC: International Life Sciences Institute, 1993).
[59] W.H. Lewis, *Technological Risk* (New York: WW Norton, 1990), 37-41.

1. Understanding the Importance of Messages

Each message may contain factual, inferential, value-oriented, and symbolic meaning.[60] While risk analysts have struggled to maintain a clear distinction between facts and values of risk management, values are reflected in how risks are characterized.[61] Scientific facts are "socially constructed in part, and ... embody innumerable biases."[62] The data are evaluated in a social, cultural, and political context, and assessments reflect political issues.[63] Experts and laypersons might agree about the fatalities that a technology causes in an average year, but still differ on how that risk is characterized or defined.

Some technical information is unwanted by members of the public. Communications should tell people what they need to know and do. Fischhoff states that "telling way more than people need to know can be (and be seen as) deliberately unhelpful."[64] Efforts to model decisionmaking by patients suggested that only a few of the possible side effects had a practical impact on agreeing to a medical procedure.[65] The implication of this is that people with little knowledge of a subject only want a few critical facts in order to make a decision. They want qualitative information on how a risk "works" and are less interested in a quantification of parameters about the risk.[66]

Technical, probabilistic models overlook some of the equity issues that are important to the general public.[67] Controversy and debate between experts widen the gap between scientific assessment and popular perception, eroding confidence in the decisionmaking process.[68] While technical risk assessment has focused narrowly on the probability of events and the magnitude of specific consequences, the public judges risk on such concepts as whether they chose to be exposed to it, whether they can control it, whether it is a newly apprehended problem, and whether it has catastrophic potential. In preparing for a pandemic it is important not only to draft messages but also to carefully consider their impact.

---

[60] H. D. Lasswell, "The Structure And Function Of Communication In Society," in L. Bryson (ed), *The Communication Of Ideas: A Series Of Addresses* (New York: Cooper Square, 1948), 32–35.

[61] B. Fischhoff, "Risk Perception And Communication Unplugged: Twenty Years Of Process," Paper for Addressing agencies' risk communication needs: a symposium to discuss next steps (Annapolis, MD: 1994); E.A.C. Crouch and R. Wilson, *Risk/Benefit Analysis* (Cambridge, MA: Ballinger, 1981).

[62] E. J. Woodhouse, "Toward More Usable Technology Policy Analyses," in G. C. Bryner, *Science, Technology and Politics* (Boulder, CO: Westview Press, 1992), 18.

[63] J. Ansell and F. Wharton, *Risk Analysis, Assessment and Management* (New York: John Wiley, 1992).

[64] Fischhoff, paper for addressing agencies' risk communication needs.

[65] J. F. Merz, B. Fischhoff, D.J. Mazur, and P.S. Fischbeck, "A Decision-Analytic Approach To Developing Standards Of Disclosure For Medical Informed Consent," *Journal of Products and Toxics Liabilities*, 1993, 15: 191–215.

[66] Fischhoff, "Risk Perception And Communication Unplugged: Twenty Years Of Process." Paper for Addressing agencies' risk communication needs: a symposium to discuss next steps (Annapolis, MD: 1994).

[67] J. M. Doderlein, "Understanding Risk Management," *Risk Analysis*, 1983, 3: 17–21; R.E. Kasperson (ed.), *Equity Issues In Radioactive Waste Management* (Cambridge, MA: Oelgeschlager, Gunn & Hain, Inc, 1983).

[68] H. J. Otway and D. von Winterfeldt, "Beyond Acceptable Risk: On The Social Acceptability Of Technologies," *Policy Sciences*, 1982, 14: 247–256.

Newly apprehended risks have "signal value" as portending a new problem or the emergence of something that is more serious than previously understood.[69] The negative imagery can confer stigma, particularly if vivid photographs drive home how bad the situation has become. So the explicit message delivered may be quite different from the implicit message heard and processed by the public. Kasperson and his colleagues note how events can be transformed in the messages that are used to describe them. An event or announcement can convey meanings that were unintended by the speaker. Using Kasperson's approach, adapted to the present case, we could envision the following hypothetical translation from explicit to inferred messages:

- Message: pandemic looms > Inference: new catastrophic risk threatens me.
- Message: case confirmed > Inference: officials cannot control the outbreak.
- Message: dispute about how well precautions work to prevent infection > Inference: experts do not understand the risk.
- Message: officials cannot treat all who are ill > Inference: officials do not care about people.
- Message: disagreement on medical treatment > Inference: officials are concealing some risks.
- Message: adverse side effects from vaccine > Inference: there's no hope.
- Message: quarantine imposed > Inference: we are trapped in an infected zone.

In such a fashion, facts are endowed with meaning when messages are conveyed. The meaning in the inferred messages may or may not accurately reflect reality (in the hypothetical above, they do not). In a study of how the West Nile Virus outbreak was handled in New York, Covello and his collaborators said that messages must be evaluated on various criteria, such as which messages:

- Are most effective.
- Are most respectful of different values and worldviews.
- Raise moral or ethical issues.
- Are most respectful of process.[70]

To that we could add the criteria of which messages are least likely to be transformed into a fearful supposition and misinterpreted by the general public. This suggests the importance of examining the capabilities of the sources—the transmitters—of risk information.

---

[69] R.E. Kasperson, O. Renn, P. Slovic, H.S. Brown, J. Emel, R. Goble, J.X. Kasperson, and S. Ratick, "The Social Amplification Of Risk: A Conceptual Framework," *Risk Analysis*, 1988, 8(2): 177-87.
[70] V. T. Covello, R. G. Peters, J. G. Wojtecki, R. C. Hyde, "Risk Communication, The West Nile Virus Epidemic, And Bioterrorism: Responding To The Communication Challenges Posed By The Intentional Or Unintentional Release Of A Pathogen In An Urban Setting," *Journal of Urban Health. Bulletin of the New York Academy of Medicine*, June 2001, 78(2): 382-391.

2. Evaluating the Credibility of the Sources of Information

Risk is amplified when official sources of information are slow, contradictory, or appear to be hiding bad news; into this vacuum flow speculation, rumors, and fear.[71] The general advice for communicators has included the following recommendations by Covello and Allen, which were distributed by the EPA:[72]

- Accept and involve the public as a legitimate partner.
- Plan carefully and evaluate your efforts. Begin with clear objectives. Aim specific messages at target groups.
- Listen to the public's concerns. Opinion research and interviews can be used.
- Be honest, frank, and open; trust and credibility are your most precious assets.
- Coordinate and collaborate with other credible parties. Communicate with trustworthy sources like scientists, physicians, university professors, and local officials.
- Meet the needs of the media.
- Speak clearly and with compassion.

Organizations are advised to carefully prepare for public announcements. Practical communication advice has included such things as being organized before making any comment as well as some of the following preparatory activities:

- Decide upon an objective before making any statement publicly. What does the spokesperson want to accomplish?
- Anticipate questions and concerns. Identify categories of concern and ask: What do people want to know?
- Decide in advance what messages to deliver. Make sure that there is a message for each category of concern (see above). Messages should be accurate and concise.
- Review the subjects that cannot be commented about. Most public relations gaffes involve inadvertent comments blurted out without much thought. While stonewalling is a bad idea, speculation, guesses, and the revealing of confidential information ought to be avoided.
- Select a main message to emphasize in a statement, interview, or press release. Carefully chosen and emphatically delivered, this message could become the newspaper quote or the TV "sound bite."
- Consider whether this main message is related positively to the objective in step one. If not, develop a better message.

Those in charge of delivering the messages sometimes complain that the public does not understand the message. The problem, however, may be miscommunication from the source. Studies of risk perception have shown that the public's fears should not be

---

[71] Powell and Leiss.
[72] V. T. Covello and F. Allen, *Seven Cardinal Rules of Risk Communication* (Washington, DC: U.S. Environmental Protection Agency, 1988).

blamed on irrationality or ignorance, but that many reactions could be attributed to sensitivity to social, psychological, and technical attributes of hazards that were not well understood by those making risk assessments and communicating the information to the public.[73] The failure of risk communication to facilitate policy solutions is attributed by Slovic to "a failure to appreciate the complex and socially determined nature of the concept *risk*."[74] This concept is subjective and value-laden, something that some communicators themselves do not seem to understand.

How the story is framed is crucial. It is now recognized that people evaluate risk of such things as surgery much differently if the same prognosis is presented in the form of mortality rather than survival rates.[75] People are more fearful hearing the odds in terms of death than the same odds stated in terms of surviving. An example of this comes from a study by McNeil and collaborators who asked people to assume they had cancer and to choose between two therapies: radiation or surgery.

One group was presented with the probabilities framed in terms of surviving for various lengths after surgery while the second group received probabilities framed in terms of dying after surgery. The odds were the same: 68 percent survived for a year and 32 percent died. When the odds were framed in terms of surviving surgery, only 18 percent chose the alternative treatment, radiation. When the identical odds were framed in terms of dying after surgery, 44 percent chose radiation instead.[76] McNeil's study showed the same results for physicians as for laypersons. This is of particular relevance to medical practitioners who must discuss alternatives for a variety of illness, including those caused by new viruses.

Because in our democracy it is not possible to exclude the public from having a role in risk management, controversies regularly occur. Better communication has not made decision making on thorny problems, such as nuclear waste, any easier. Slovic attributes the shortcomings not to poor communication but to lack of trust in the sources of information. If the risk manager is trusted, communication is relatively simple, but if trust is diminished, communication cannot bridge the gap.[77] He notes the following difficulties for those who want to be trusted:

- Trust is easier to destroy than create.
- Negative events that diminish trust are more noticeable than trust-building efforts.
- Trust-destroying events carry greater weight with the public than positive events.
- Bad news is seen as more believable than good news.

---

[73] P. Slovic, "Perceived Risk, Trust And Democracy," *Risk Analysis,* 1993, 13: 675–682.

[74] P. Slovic, "Trust, Emotion, Sex, Politics and Science; Surveying the Risk-Assessment Battlefield," in M. H. Bazerman, D. M. Messick, A. E. Tenbrunsel, and K. A. Wade-Benzoni (eds), *Environment, Ethics, and Behavior* (San Francisco, CA: New Lexington, 1997), 277–313.

[75] A. Tversky and D. Kahneman, "The Framing Of Decisions And The Psychology Of Choice," *Science,* 1981, 211: 453–458.

[76] B. J. McNeil, S. G. Puaker, H. C. Sox, Jr and A. Tversky, "On The Elicitation Of Preferences For Alternative Therapies," *New England Journal of Medicine,* 1982, 306(21): 1259-1262.

[77] J. Fessenden-Raden, J.M. Fitchen, and J.S. Heath, "Providing Risk Information In Communities: Factors Influencing What Is Heard And Accepted," *Science Technology and Human Values,* 1987, 12: 94-101.

- Distrust, once initiated, reinforces and perpetuates distrust.
- Distrust colors interpretations of events, reinforcing prior belief.
- Once trust is lost, it may take a long time to regain it.[78]

Lack of trust has been identified as an important factor in divisive environmental health controversies. Lack of trust is a major reason why the public often rejects scientists' risk assessments.[79] Obviously, trust should be established in advance of a problem and nurtured before a health crisis. Environmental case studies, such as the chemical industry's Responsible Care Program, show that proactive community outreach is one of the best ways to achieve this goal.[80] In environmental controversies, citizen advisory panels have been effective in gaining constructive public participation and might be of utility in coping with the threat of bioterrorism.[81] People want to be treated with respect, and they want to be leveled with; "people fear that those who disrespect them are also disenfranchising them."[82] One communication skill helpful in building trust is listening rather than speaking.

3. Understanding the Importance of Mass Media

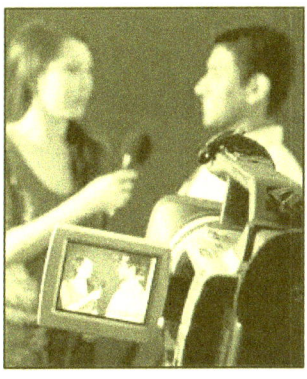

Communicating via the media poses the risk of being misunderstood, taken out of context, distrusted, and sometimes distorted.

It is important to recognize that journalists are always in a hurry. They are competitive, and peer group pressure is intense. Reporters consistently compare stories after they appear. Information has to be compressed and oversimplified, and the news must be interesting. More often than not, reporters are not specialists in all the fields they cover. Furthermore, the press is dependent upon sources, which makes them subject to manipulation. Given these pressures, it is not surprising that news stories often include inaccurate information; what is more surprising is how often they hit the mark. Part of the problem in working with the press to communicate a message stems from four related shortcomings in journalism:[83]

[78] P. Slovic, "Perceived Risk, Trust and Democracy," *Risk Analysis,* 1993, 13: 675-682.

[79] P. Slovic, *The Perception of Risk* (Sterling, VA: Earthscan, 2000).

[80] V. T. Covello, et al, "Risk communication, the West Nile Virus epidemic;" S. Santos, V. T. Covello, D. B. McCallum, "Industry response to SARA Title III: Pollution Prevention, Risk Reduction, and Risk Communication," *Risk Analysis,* 1996, 16(1): 57--65.

[81] F. M. Lynn and G. J. Busenberg, "Citizen Advisory Committees and Environmental Policy: What We Know, What's Left to Discover," *Risk Analysis,* 1005, 15(2): 147-161.

[82] Fischhoff, paper for addressing agencies' risk communication needs.

[83] F. Rowan, *Broadcast Fairness: Doctrine Practice, Prospects* (New York: Longman, 1984), 124-129.

- Much news coverage is superficial. This is because most journalists are generalists, and most know a little about a lot of things. It is often a general assignment reporter, rather than a specialist, who frames the first story about an issue.

- Much news coverage is sensationalistic. Media overkill is apparent in major disasters. Most reporters resist the temptation to exaggerate or hype stories, but the temptation is always present in a business that depends upon ratings and circulation for revenue.

- Subjectivity or bias is inherent. Every person is a subjective creature. We are all captives of our own mindset, worldview, the values imparted by parents, taught by schools, learned with peers, conditioned on the job, watched on TV and the like. The bias is best understood, not in familiar liberal versus conservative terms, but as an overarching skepticism, a negative attitude about large institutions, leaders, and public officials. This skepticism can have profound consequences when reporters are called to cover government statements about risk, safety, and disaster.

- Clear and enforceable standards do not exist in journalism. Given our First Amendment, reporters are burdened with almost no external checks and balances. Very few professions have such ill-defined ethical guidelines with so few sanctions for violations. The lack of accountability makes deviance from standards possible.

The result of these perils—superficiality, sensationalism, subjectivity, and lack of standards—is that those who want to communicate via the media are at risk of being misunderstood, taken out of context, distrusted and—rarely, but sometimes—distorted. The nature of journalism makes possible exaggerated, dramatic portrayals of major issues.

Some risks have been greatly amplified by news media coverage. For example, the chemical leak in Bhopal, India, which claimed thousands of lives, the destruction of the *Challenger* and *Columbia* spacecraft, the nuclear accidents at Three Mile Island and Chernobyl, the *Exxon Valdez* oil spill, the adulteration of Tylenol capsules with cyanide, the "mad cow" (BSE) controversy in the United Kingdom all represent cases that have been amplified in the media. Affect-laden messages (of dread, catastrophic impact, unfairness, and loss of control) exaggerate risks associated with nuclear and chemical technologies.[84] News media coverage of risk makes it more difficult to get a proper perspective on risks. Risks from dramatic and sensational causes of death—accidents, homicides, natural disasters—tend to be overstated, while non-dramatic causes—asthma, emphysema, diabetes—tend to be underestimated.[85]

---

[84] E. Peters and P. Slovic, "The Role of Affect and Worldviews as Orienting Dispositions in the Perception and Acceptance of Nuclear Power," *Journal of Applied Social Psychology,* 1996, 26: 1427-1453.

[85] S. Lichtenstein, P. Slovic, B. Fischhoff, M. Layman, and B. Combs, "Judged Frequency of Lethal Events," *Journal of Experimental Psychology,* 1978, 79: 236-240; M. G. Morgan, P. Slovic, I. Nair, D. Geisler, D. G. MacGregor, B. Fischhoff, D. Lincoln and K. Florig, "Powerline Frequency Electric and Magnetic Fields: A Pilot Study of Risk Perception," *Risk Analysis,* 1985, 5: 139-149.

No matter how balanced the news coverage, reassuring claims do not have the power of fear-arousing messages.[86] Because the news media tend to give disproportionate attention to dramatic, unusual (rare) risks, it is not surprising that popular estimates of leading causes of death are related to the amount of media coverage they get.[87] A controlled study by Johnson and Tversky found that reading a story about one type of fatal event, such as leukemia, homicide, or fire, increased the perceived frequencies for all hazards.[88] In other words, bad news arouses negative affect, which has a general influence on perception, beyond the specific risk. Thus, media coverage might have a pervasive and subtle effect on overall perceptions of risk, making the world seem very unsafe.[89]

4. Understanding How the Public Receives Risk Information

The psychologist Seymour Epstein has noted that in everyday life "people apprehend reality in two fundamentally different ways, one variously labeled intuitive, automatic, natural, non-verbal, narrative, and experimental, and the other analytical, deliberative, verbal, and rational."[90] It would be erroneous to conclude that lay perceptions of risk are all derived from emotion; affective processes interact with reason in all normal thinking.[91] In general, people are haphazard in accumulating information. People tend to extrapolate from events they learn about. For instance, Johnson and Tversky found that people who read in the newspaper about a tragic death tended to exaggerate how often such deaths occurred.[92] The tendency for people to increase their frequency estimates for causes of death learned from the news media could be a problem in a health controversy as stories about casualties reinforce alarm.

Anthropologists use the term "indigenous technical knowledge" when referring to how a non-expert layperson understands how his or her world works.[93] People tend to employ rules of thumb in making decisions, and these are susceptible to biases, misconceptions, and illusions of validity.[94] Popular judgments about uncertainty rely on simple cognitive rules of thumb, which result in error.[95] The picture is not entirely bleak. "One of the

[86] J. Sorensen, J. Soderstrom, E. Copenhaver, S. Carnes, and R. Bolin, *Impacts of Hazardous Technology: The Psycho-social Effects of Restarting TMI-1,* L. W. Milbrath (ed), SUNY Series in Environmental Public Policy (Albany: State University of New York Press, 1987).
[87] B. Combs and P. Slovic, "Newspaper Coverage of Causes of Death," *Journalism Quarterly,* 1979, 56(4): 837-843, 849.
[88] E. J. Johnson and A. Tversky, "Affect, Generalization, and the Perception of Risk," *Journal of Personality and Social Psychology,* 1983, 45: 20-31
[89] Slovic, *The Perception of Risk.*
[90] S. Epstein, "Integration of the Cognitive and the Psychodynamic Unconscious," *American Psychologist*; 1994, 49: 710.
[91] Slovic, *Perception of Risk*; A. R. Damasio, *Descartes Error: Emotion, Reason, and the Human Brain* (New York: Avon, 1994).
[92] E. J. Johnson and A. Tversky, "Affect, Generalization, and the Perception of Risk," *Journal of Personality and Social Psychology,* 1983, 45: 20–31.
[93] D. W. Brokensha, D. M. Warren and O. Werner, O, *Indigenous Knowledge: Systems and Development* (Lanham, MD: University Press of America, 1980).
[94] D. Kahneman, P. Slovic and A. Tversky (eds), *Judgment Under Uncertainty; Heuristics and Biases* (New York: Cambridge University Press, 1982).
[95] M. G. Morgan and M. Henrion, *Uncertainty: A Guide to Dealing with Uncertainty in Quantitative Risk and Policy Analysis* (New York: Cambridge University Press, 1990).

miracles of democratic life is the ability of lay people, often with little formal education, to master technical material when sufficiently motivated," according to Fischhoff. "Unfortunately for risk managers, the motivation for this self-education often comes from a feeling of having been wronged."[96]

Relatively small risks can be magnified if they seem to portend broader social impact or potential catastrophic harm in the future.[97] A thorough discussion about risk may not calm people's anxiety if social or ideological concerns predominate. Hidden agendas need to be examined in the open.[98] Attributes not grounded in the actual danger influence the perception of risk. For instance, stigmatization of certain risks, like nuclear waste, AIDS, or some forms of mental illness, increases the negative perception of those risks.[99] If fear grows about a contagious disease, it is likely that infected persons will feel stigmatized as others shun them.

To address such political and social factors, improved methods of risk management include negotiation, mediation, public oversight, and citizen involvement.[100] Public participation can lead to more successful ways to manage risk. Activities that engage stakeholders in dialogue about resolving disputes and building trust are worthwhile efforts aimed at reaching consensus.[101] How many community leaders have been involved in planning about quarantine in the event of a pandemic, bioterror attack, or other health emergency? Have citizen groups been asked to evaluate the specific advice on how individuals can protect themselves and their families from the risk of avian influenza? Have civic leaders been asked how medical triage should work—and what standards should be employed—if facilities were overwhelmed?

In sum, the research into risk communication shows that no theory has yet answered all the questions about why people perceive risks the way they do. It has offered practical guidance on ways to communicate—or more precisely, mistakes to avoid while communicating. It is now widely recognized that poor risk communication could cause fear and poor decisions by individuals and agencies alike. To mitigate such problems in a future pandemic, it would be wise to have a collaborative process to improve decision making, develop messages, build credibility for official sources, deal more openly and effectively with the media, and carefully consider how best to help people understand what they can do to empower and protect themselves.

---

[96] Fischhoff, "Risk Perception And Communication Unplugged: Twenty Years Of Process," Paper for Addressing agencies' risk communication needs: a symposium to discuss next steps (Annapolis, MD: 1994).

[97] P. Slovic, B. Fischhoff, and S. Lichtenstein, "Modeling the Societal Impact of Fatal Accidents," *Management Science*, 1984, 30: 464-474.

[98] Edwards and von Winterfeldt.

[99] Slovic, *The Perception of Risk.*

[100] NRC, Committee on Risk Characterization, *Understanding risk: Informing Decisions in a Democratic Society,* P. C. Stern and H. V. Fineberg (eds) (Washington, DC: National Academy Press, 1996).

[101] M. G. Morgan, B. Fischhoff, A. Bostrom, L. Lave, C. J. Atman, "Communicating Risk to the Public," *Environmental Science and Technology,* 1992, 26(11): 2048-2056.

Your Organization, Your Plan

Writing Your Plan

The odds are that your organization is not prepared for a pandemic. A report released in May 2006 noted that 68 percent of companies with $1 billion in revenue are *not* ready for a pandemic.[102] For the fiscal year ending April 2006, bird flu was only mentioned 388 times in annual and quarterly reports, according to filings with the Securities and Exchange Commission.[103] Typical of those who have thought about it is the comment made by George Chizmar, vice president of IT at Apple Vacations in Newton Square, PA: "We have our hurricane playbook as far as contingency planning goes, and we'd probably amend that for bird flu."[104]

This is not just another hurricane. Hurricanes and other natural disasters are usually constrained in time and space. Additionally, infrastructure damage usually accompanies the event. A flu pandemic, by definition, will be worldwide. Previous pandemics have had "waves" of increased illness and death. The 1918 pandemic lasted 18 months, with three distinct peaks of increased morbidity and mortality. Thus, the response to a pandemic will be distinctly different from the response to a singular, catastrophic event.

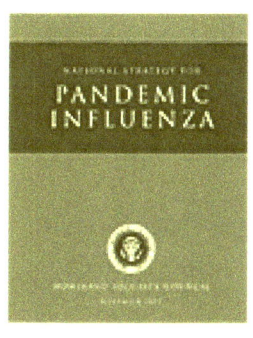

In November 2005, the Federal Government released its National Strategy for Pandemic Influenza.[105] It can be viewed as a military plan and interpreted as the "commander's intent." That is, it describes large goals, or end-states, while deliberately not providing the detail as to how to accomplish them. In large measure, the details are left to planners at lower levels. The plan identifies the responsibilities of the Federal Government, States and Localities, the Private Sector and Critical Infrastructure Entities, and Individuals and Families.

National Strategy for
Pandemic Influenza,
November 2005.
Available at:
http://www.whitehouse.gov/homeland/nspi.pdf

---

[102] EWeek.com, "The Pandemic Plan: Wing It," May 8, 2006. Print Archives, vol.23, no. 19.
[103] Ibid.
[104] Ibid.
[105] See <http://www.whitehouse.gov/homeland/pandemic-influenza.html>.

Federal Government Responsibilities

- Advancing international preparedness, surveillance, response, and containment activities.
- Supporting the establishment of countermeasure stockpiles and production capacity.
- Ensuring that Federal departments and agencies, including Federal health care systems, have developed and exercised preparedness and response plans that take into account the potential impact of a pandemic on the Federal workforce and are configured to support state, local, and private sector efforts as appropriate.
- Facilitating state and local planning through funding and guidance.
- Providing guidance to the private and public sectors on preparedness and response planning, in conjunction with states and communities.

States and Localities Responsibilities

- Ensuring that all reasonable measures are taken to limit the spread of an outbreak within and beyond the community's borders.
- Establishing comprehensive and credible preparedness and response plans that are exercised on a regular basis.
- Integrating non-health entities in the planning for a pandemic, including law enforcement, utilities, city services, and political leadership.
- Establishing state- and community-based stockpiles and distribution systems to support a comprehensive pandemic response.
- Identifying key spokespersons for the community and ensuring that they are educated in risk communication and have coordinated crisis communications plans.
- Providing public education campaigns on pandemic influenza and public and private interventions.

The Private Sector and Critical Infrastructure Entities

- Establishing an ethic of infection control in the workplace that is reinforced during the annual influenza season, to include, if possible, options for working offsite while ill, systems to reduce infection transmission, and worker education.
- Establishing contingency systems to maintain delivery of essential goods and services during times of significant and sustained worker absenteeism.
- Where possible, establishing mechanisms to allow workers to provide services from home if public health officials advise against non-essential travel outside the home.
- Establishing partnerships with other members of the private sector to provide mutual support and maintenance of essential services during a pandemic.

Individuals and Families

- Taking precautions to prevent the spread of infection to others if an individual or a family member has symptoms of influenza.
- Being prepared to follow public health guidance, which may include limitation of attendance at public gatherings and non-essential travel for several days or weeks.
- Keeping supplies of materials at home, as recommended by authorities, to support essential needs of the household for several days, if necessary.

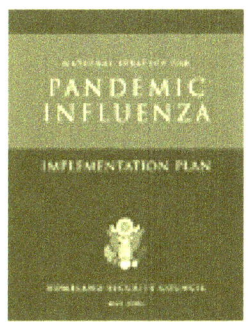

In May 2006, the Federal government released the Implementation Plan for the National Strategy.[106] The report provided detailed direction for all stakeholders—government at all levels, the private sector, and private individuals—across the following six functional areas:

Implementation Plan for the
National Strategy, May 2006.
Available at:
http://www.whitehouse.gov/homeland/nspi_implementation.pdf

- International Efforts—prevent and contain outbreaks abroad.
- Transportation and Borders—slow the arrival and spread of a pandemic.
- Protecting Human Health—limit spread and mitigate illness.
- Protecting Animal Health—control influenza with human pandemic potential in animals.
- Law Enforcement, Public Safety, and Security—ensure civil order during a pandemic.
- Planning by Institutions—protect personnel and ensure continuity of operations.

The implementation plan further identifies four priority actions for the Federal Government:

- Advance international capacity for early warning and response.
- Limit the arrival and spread of a pandemic.
- Provide clear guidance to all stakeholders.
- Accelerate the development of countermeasures.

The implementation plan also underscored the importance of preparedness by individuals, communities, and the private sector by specifically noting the following:

---

[106] See <http://www.whitehouse.gov/homeland/nspi_implementation.pdf>.

- *Individuals Must Actively Participate.* Simple infection-control measures, including hand washing and staying home when ill, are critical. Individuals should actively participate in their communities' responses.
- *State and Local Governments Must Prepare.* Pandemics are global events, but individual communities experience pandemics as local events. State and local governments, with clear guidance from the Federal Government, should be prepared to implement community-wide measures, such as school closures and suspension of public gatherings, to halt the spread of disease.
- *The Private Sector Must Prepare.* The private sector, with targeted and timely guidance from the Federal Government, should develop plans to provide essential services, even in the face of sustained and significant absenteeism. Businesses should also integrate their planning into community planning.

A May 22, 2006 article noted that local municipalities were criticizing the Federal Government for a lack of guidance and resources. The Department of Health and Human Services (HHS) responded by saying that HHS had been stressing for some time that cities and states should not rely on Federal resources. Unlike hurricanes, a pandemic could erupt in many regions of the country simultaneously, overloading Federal resources. Patrick Libbey, the executive director of the National Association of County and City Health Officials summed it up best when he noted that, "Ultimately, preparedness happens at the local level . . . the actual planning and implementation cannot be directed from Washington or state capitols."[107]

That is the thrust of this document. While Libbey was speaking specifically about plans for dealing with health-related aspects of a pandemic, his comments are equally true for continuity of operations planning.

Appendix 1 lists websites that provide pandemic plans or guidance for writing a plan. Some of the websites listed offer generic information. However, the purpose of this paper is to provide as much specificity as possible. Thus, many of the websites that were reviewed were not included, as they lacked specificity to a given sector. Where possible, we have gathered websites that address plans for a given sector—business, schools, government, and others. Some are health related and concern how organizations will respond *to* the flu, rather than how they will conduct their usual business *during* the flu. While responding to the flu is important, the focus of your organizational plan should be on conducting business during the flu.

In reviewing a number of plans, it was noted that many organizations were essentially placing their name on a coversheet and using a plan developed by another organization. In this context, plagiarism is *not* a crime! That is not the point. The point is that the plans were inappropriate for the organizations—one size does not fit all. In preparing a plan for your organization, leaders should consider all of the factors discussed in this paper, review the plans at the various websites, and then create the plan that works best for your own organization.

---

[107] Congressional Quarterly, May 22, 2006. Available online at <http://www.cq.com/displayweekly.do?issue=20060522>.

Testing Your Plan

Writing the plan is only part of the effort. Testing your plan is vital so that weaknesses and inconsistencies can be identified as early as possible. The first step in testing is to conduct a "table-top exercise."[108] These exercises are fairly inexpensive to conduct and give a good "first-cut" analysis of your plan's strengths and weaknesses. With a table-top exercise, the real desire is to see where points of friction might exist. Do the various pieces fit together?

Start with a reasonable scenario. Many public health/emergency response exercises have underlying assumptions in the scenario that are simply unrealistic. This is particularly true when the scenario involves the spread of disease. All too often, scenarios over-estimate the rate of spread and/or the degree of morbidity and mortality, and the exercise comes to an early halt because all systems are overwhelmed.

It is better to start with an unrealistically optimistic set of assumptions than to start with overly pessimistic ones. The purpose of the first attempts at a table-top exercise is not to see if your plan is ready for a pandemic. The purpose is to identify points of friction. Does the plan allow for good communication between different players? Does the plan identify all of the players needed for your situation?

Additionally, by starting with a modest scenario, senior-level people from your organization will not need to be involved with the first attempt to use the plan. Exercise the plan using the people who prepared it and identify the points of friction and correct them. After this is done, plan an exercise that involves the organization's senior staff. Depending on your organization's budget and size, a table-top exercise may be sufficient to help evaluate preparedness for pandemic flu. Or, it may lead to a larger exercise that involves other organizations and/or a greater number of players from your organization. Again, every time improvements are made to the plan, consider running a table-top exercise to test the improvements before staging a large exercise or one involving senior staff.

Additional Considerations

In addition to the numerous concerns about the mental health of the workforce and the physical setting of the workspace, other tasks should be considered when preparing for a pandemic.

The Workload: It is hard to predict what the effect will be on your organization's actual workload. In health care, the workload likely will increase. In the travel industry, the workload may decline. In secondary education, the workload may stay the same, but the venue may change—greater use of the Internet and media, for example.

---

[108] The Department of Health and Human Services offers a Pandemic Influenza Tabletop Exercise Package at <http://www.hhs.gov/nvpo/pandemics/tabletopex.html>.

Conduct an analysis of the tasks that are required for your organization to continue operating and prioritize them. Concentrate on ensuring that those tasks labeled as "mission essential" can be met, even if only half of your staff is available. Begin cross-training employees, so everyone is familiar with the mission essential tasks and can perform them, if necessary. Identify those tasks that can be done remotely—via the Internet—and establish secure websites.

Proportionate Absenteeism: If your organization's work can be accomplished over the Internet, then office absenteeism does not necessarily mean 8 hours of work will be lost for each absent employee. Some workers will be home sick. Obviously, they will be unavailable for work. Some workers will be well but needed at home to care for those who are sick. Depending upon the circumstances—severity of illness, number of ill, etc.—an absent employee may be able to complete a few hours of work during a day. Some workers will be well, but unavailable due to fear or the need to care for children out of school. They may be available for a full, or least a partial, day's work. The hours of availability may not be during the normal working hours, but the work could still be completed. Additionally, feeling connected to a normal part of life will likely be conducive to maintaining the mental health of employees.

24-Hours a Day: If possible, establish a 24-hour work cycle. By moving to 8-hour shifts, the number of people at your workplace could be cut to one-third, significantly aiding the effort to establish social distancing. Additionally, those people who are absent could be more easily integrated into such a cycle and their work timed to fit into the overall flow of your organization's work.

Establish Help Lines: Identify phone lines and numbers that will be dedicated to employee help lines. Identify those individuals who will work the help lines and begin training them now. Establish the help lines at the lowest possible level—that is, each distinct group within your organization would have a specific number to call, and the group members would know the person answering the phone. (This is an example of a task that could easily be done remotely by an employee at home.) One organizational helpline with a recorded message would not be conducive to providing trusted, credible information.

Review Personnel Policies: There may be legal or regulatory implications to your plan. Those need to be reviewed now. In addition, all of your workforce will need to fully understand policies on leave and telecommuting. Even if your pandemic plan does not require changing any of your current policies, it would be a good time to review them with your organization's members.

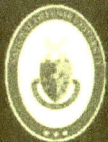
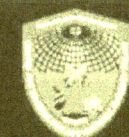

BIRD FLU AND YOU

**Prepared by: Robert Armstrong, PhD[1] and Stephen Prior, PhD[2] with Natalie Tedder, BS[3],
Mary Beth Hill-Harmon, MSPH[4], and Nicki Borkowski, MS[5]**

Four Simple Things You Can Do To Protect Yourself And Your Family

COVER YOUR COUGH AND SNEEZE

- Cover your mouth and nose with a tissue
- Put your tissue in the trash can
- If you do not have a tissue, cough or sneeze into your upper sleeve, not your hands

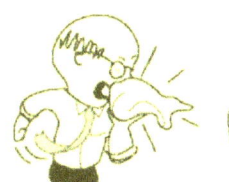
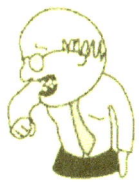

WASH YOUR HANDS

- Wash hands with warm, soapy water for at least 10-15 seconds OR use a hand sanitizer after:
  - Coughing or sneezing
  - Using the bathroom
  - Caring for a sick person
  - Handling garbage or animal waste

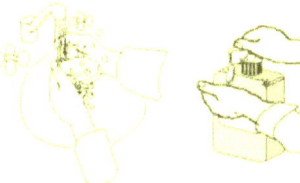

KEEP LIVING AND WORK AREAS CLEAN

- Clean areas with household detergents (dishwashing liquid, laundry detergent, hand soap)
- Sanitize surfaces with bleach or alcohol

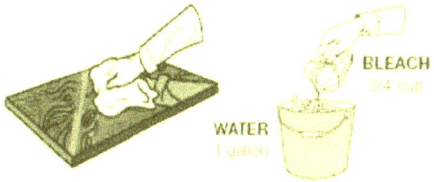

BLEACH
1/4 cup

WATER
1 gallon

KEEP YOUR DISTANCE

- Avoid crowds
- Limit your travel
- Travel to and from work during off-peak hours, if possible
- Work from home, if possible

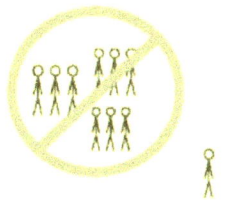
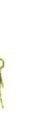

There are many common sense, non-medical steps you can take to protect yourself, your coworkers and your loved ones. Following these procedures can significantly limit the spread of the virus—both H5N1 and the virus causing seasonal flu.

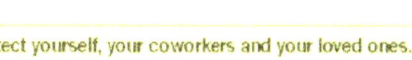

Cleaning and Sterilizing:	Sterilizing Agents	Recommended Use	Precautions
	Household (Laundry) Bleach		
	Rubbing Alcohol		

Keep bleach and rubbing alcohol away from children.

Do not drink bleach or rubbing alcohol.

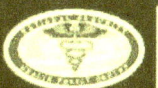

AUGUST 2006 v1.0

Appendix 1: Getting Started

This appendix contains a collection of websites that may provide helpful information and guidance to your organization, as you complete your particular COOP plan. No one plan listed will fit the specific needs of your particular organization. The websites are organized by sector (business, education, government, etc.) but you will likely find useful information in all of them. Take what is of use for your organization and develop the rest of your plan to fit your organization's unique requirements.

Helpful Websites for Developing Your COOP Plan

Business
http://www.hram.org/downloads/Business%20Continuity%20Planning%20For%20An%20Influenza%20Pandemic.pdf
http://www.fcchamber.org/data/pandemicplan2.pdf
http://www.cme-mec.ca/pdf/CME_Pandemic_Guide.pdf
http://healthcareproviders.org.nz/publication/documents/ExampleofaNZPandemicManagementPlan.DOC
http://healthcareproviders.org.nz/publication/important-documents.htm
http://www.idph.state.ia.us/pandemic/common/pdf/planning_guide.pdf
http://sev.prnewswire.com/computer-electronics/20060404/LATU05104042006-1.html
http://www.med.govt.nz/upload/27552/planning-guide.pdf
http://www.interaction.org/files.cgi/5259_IA_Pandemic_Continuity_Plan_PUBLIC.pdf
http://www.aamp.com/documents/AIPandemicImpact.pdf
Education
http://www.cshema.org/resource/ACHA%20Pandemic%20guide%20rev_3.doc
http://lime.weeg.uiowa.edu/~provost//docs/pandemic.pdf
http://www.oseh.umich.edu/buscont/Business%20Continuity%20Planning%20-%20Pandemic%20Disease%20Scenario%20Guideline.pdf
http://www.ahc.umn.edu/img/assets/19701/Pandemic_Influenza_Preparedness_Workplan_121505.pdf
http://www.ahc.umn.edu/img/assets/19701/PandemicInfluenzaHousingPlan070506PhoneNumbersRemoved.pdf
http://ehs.unc.edu/healthy/template.doc http://ehs.unc.edu/healthy/coop.shtml
http://www.sfsu.edu/~hrwww/risk_mgmt/bcp/bcp_obj_mile.pdf
Federal Government
http://training.fema.gov/EMIWeb/downloads/COOPLessonSummary.pdf
http://www.pandemicflu.gov
http://www.opm.gov/pandemic/
Financial
http://www.rbnz.govt.nz/crisismgmt/2198851.pdf
Hospitals/Health Care Facilities
http://www.hhs.gov/pandemicflu/plan/sup3.html
http://www.state.nj.us/health/flu/documents/influenza_plan.pdf
http://www.psnc.org.uk/uploaded_txt/ServiceContinuityPlanningforpharmacyguidance.pdf
http://www.aspenrha.com/images/stories/pdf/pandemic/pandemic_overview.pdf
http://mass.gov/dph/bioterrorism/advisorygrps/word_files/hospital_coop_11_05.doc
Local Government
http://mkcclegisearch.metrokc.gov/attachments/20144.doc
http://www.sfcdcp.org/UserFiles/File/InfectiousDiseasesAtoZ/City_Agency._Pan_Flu_Continuity_Plan.6.19.06.pdf
http://www.santarosa.fl.gov/emergency/documents/pandemicfluplan06.pdf
Public Health Departments
http://www.mahb.org/emergencyprep/COOP.doc
http://horrycounty.redcross.org/panflu/PICOOP_Guide.doc

Table A1-1

Appendix 1: Getting Started

Following is a short synopsis of the websites listed in Table A1-1.

Business

Baird Holm LLP, Business Continuity Planning for an Influenza Pandemic
This presentation focuses on how employers should prepare for a pandemic. Thought
provoking questions are laid out for business management to consider when developing
their specific COOP plan.

http://www.hram.org/downloads/Business%20Continuity%20Planning%20For%20An%2
0Influenza%20Pandemic.pdf

British Columbia Pandemic Influenza Preparedness Plan
The British Columbia Ministry of Health prepared this guide to encourage businesses to
take practical actions to manage pandemic influenza and its consequences. It applies the
principles of risk management to help businesses of all types and sizes to ensure
continuity of operations, maintain essential services, and help employees and
communities cope with illness and its impacts. Guide objectives include the following:

- Get Organized.
- Assess the Risks.
- Protect Employee Health.
- Prepare Employee Policies.
- Plan for Business Continuity.
- Prepare for Supply and Service Interruptions.
- Prepare to Fill Vacancies.
- Inform Employees.
- Inform Other Stakeholders.
- Prepare a Pandemic Influenza Management Plan.

http://www.fcchamber.org/data/pandemicplan2.pdf

Influenza Pandemic: Continuity Planning for Canadian Business
This guide is designed to help businesses minimize the risk that an influenza pandemic
poses to the health and safety of employees, the continuity of business operations, and
their bottom line. It is intended to provide all businesses in Canada with the basic
information they require in preparing continuity plans to mitigate the potential effects of
a pandemic. The guide contains the following:

- A background summary of the potential impacts of an influenza pandemic on
  business.
- An overview of the human resource issues involved.

- The critical elements that should be incorporated into business continuity strategies for managing the impact of an influenza pandemic, including how to:
    o Maintain essential activities.
    o Contain/minimize the spread of infection in the workplace.

http://www.cme-mec.ca/pdf/CME_Pandemic_Guide.pdf

New Zealand Workplace Influenza Pandemic Health Plan
This is an example of a recent pandemic health management plan that was prepared by The Shell Company Australia Limited (Shell) for use in its installations in Oceania.
The plan aims to manage the impact of influenza pandemic on employees and business via the health impacts on two main strategies:

- Containment of the disease by reducing spread within Business Facilities.
- Maintenance of essential services if containment is not possible.

http://healthcareproviders.org.nz/publication/documents/ExampleofaNZPandemicManag ementPlan.DOC

Pandemic Flu Planning Guide for Infrastructure Providers (v9 Planning Guide)
This planning guide sets out a range of information aimed primarily at companies that provide infrastructure services in the energy, communications, transport, and water and waste sectors that may be helpful in planning for the impact of a possible influenza pandemic on their employees and business.

http://healthcareproviders.org.nz/publication/important-documents.htm

Pandemic Influenza Planning Guide for Iowa Businesses
Published in January 2006 by the Iowa Department of Public Health, this guide is to assist in managing the impact of an influenza pandemic on employees and businesses based on two main strategies: reducing the spread of the virus within business facilities and sustaining essential services. The guide provides recommendations for businesses to develop a pandemic plan including the following:

- Communication to business from external or internal sources regarding the pandemic virus.
- Activities to reduce the spread of the virus.
- Social distancing (reducing person-to-person interactions by postponing conferences, conducting telephone meetings, and other activities).
- Educating employees to reduce concern.
- Handling employees who become ill at work.
- Maintenance of essential business activities.
- Identification of essential people and business functions.
- Planning for absenteeism and supplier disruption.

http://www.idph.state.ia.us/pandemic/common/pdf/planning_guide.pdf

VIACK Corporation
This company has developed a COOP guide that covers COOP plan basics, key components for an effective plan, incorporating teleworking and assessing effectiveness and results. This is not a plan for VIACK but a consulting guide for business to create a COOP.

http://sev.prnewswire.com/computer-electronics/20060404/LATU05104042006-1.html

Influenza Pandemic Planning: Business Continuity Planning Guide October 2005 (New Zealand)
This planning guide sets out a range of information aimed at New Zealand's businesses and other organizations that will be helpful in planning for the impact of a pandemic influenza on their businesses and employees. This guide was assembled to promote good workplace practices in planning for a possible pandemic.

http://www.med.govt.nz/upload/27552/planning-guide.pdf

InterAction: Pandemic Flu Continuity of Operations Plan
This plan is divided by WHO Pandemic Phases. While primarily designed to plan for the eventuality of a Phase 6 pandemic, the COOP plan is also meant to serve as a detailed checklist of all actions necessary by InterAction to prepare prior to a pandemic.

http://www.interaction.org/files.cgi/5259_IA_Pandemic_Continuity_Plan_PUBLIC.pdf

Business Continuity Planning for Meat and Poultry Processing Sector in Relation to Potential Flu Pandemic
Specific questions and issues need to be addressed in developing a Meat and Poultry COOP. This document is not meant to capture the science or policies surrounding avian influenza, but rather to provoke thought into the areas of business impact and continuity during a pandemic by asking questions that should generate discussions within individual companies. These questions are not all inclusive, but represent questions that have been developed in response to public forums where business impact and continuity have been discussed.

http://www.aamp.com/documents/AIPandemicImpact.pdf

Education

American College Health Association Pandemic Planning Guidelines
The purpose of these guidelines is to prompt college health professionals to develop pandemic preparedness plans for their campus. This document is not intended to offer detailed information about the nature of viruses nor H5N1, but rather to assist college health professionals in engaging in thoughtful discourse with partners on their campus in

the formulation of a flexible, adaptive response plan that is tailored to the needs and resources of the institution. The first part of this document offers an overview of the pandemic threat, the importance of pandemic preparedness planning, and how to get started. The second part addresses planning for a broader campus-wide response.

http://www.cshema.org/resource/ACHA%20Pandemic%20guide%20rev_3.doc

University of Iowa Pandemic Response Plan

The purpose of this plan is to provide an organized, comprehensive statement of the University's intended response to a possible influenza pandemic. The plan also serves as a written agreement among all parties to take action in the event of such an emergency and identifies emergency response organizations, facilities, and other resources that can be utilized during a public health emergency.

http://lime.weeg.uiowa.edu/~provost//docs/pandemic.pdf

University of Michigan Business Continuity Planning: Pandemic Disease Scenario

This guidance is issued by the Department of Occupational Safety and Environmental Health to provide guidance and consistency in business continuity planning for the business and finance units of the University to deal with a pandemic disease scenario.

http://www.oseh.umich.edu/buscont/Business%20Continuity%20Planning%20-%20Pandemic%20Disease%20Scenario%20Guideline.pdf

University of Minnesota Pandemic Influenza Preparedness Work Plan

The University of Minnesota developed and hosted a pandemic influenza tabletop exercise to explore the unique challenges faced in the university campus setting and to further refine the respective response roles of the University, state health department, local health departments, and the University of Minnesota Medical Center. From this, a preparedness work plan was developed that is broken down into ten areas based upon the exercise and a review of Federal guidelines:

- International Travel.
- Targeted Vaccine Distribution.
- Essential Personnel, Operations, and Services.
- Surveillance and Case Investigation.
- Healthcare Needs.
- Student Housing Needs.
- Communications.
- Internal Coordination.
- External Coordination.
- Providing Service to the Broader Community.

http://www.ahc.umn.edu/img/assets/19701/Pandemic_Influenza_Preparedness_Workplan_121505.pdf

University of Minnesota: Twin Cities Campus: Housing and Residential Life and University Dining Services Pandemic Influenza Response Plan
This plan prepares the Housing and Residential Life (HRL) and University Dining Services (UDS) to meet the housing and dining needs of students, staff, and faculty in the event of an influenza pandemic. In the event of an influenza pandemic, Housing and Residential Life and University Dining Services will have detailed specific action tasks that will be implemented in a pandemic, including establishing a Department Operations Center (DOC).

http://www.ahc.umn.edu/img/assets/19701/PandemicInfluenzaHousingPlan070506Phone
NumbersRemoved.pdf

University of North Carolina Chapel Hill Pandemic Influenza Continuity of Operations Plan
All UNC departments and units are required to use this form to complete a Continuity of Operations Plan to describe how they will operate during an influenza pandemic and afterward recover to be fully operational. This plan encourages departments to augment this template to meet their individual needs.

http://ehs.unc.edu/healthy/template.doc
In addition the University has an operational planning website:
http://ehs.unc.edu/healthy/coop.shtml

San Francisco State University Business Continuity Plan: Pandemic Objectives and Milestones
The plan outlines the paramount demand for participation in emergency planning, personal and family preparations, pandemic hygiene, and communication with colleagues and supervisors concerning health status, and monitoring of the University website.

http://www.sfsu.edu/~hrwww/risk_mgmt/bcp/bcp_obj_mile.pdf

Federal Government

FEMA COOP Federal Initiative: COOP Web-based Course
This web-based course is designed to ensure that Executive Branch departments and agencies can continue to perform their essential functions under a broad range of circumstances. This web-based lesson includes:

- What COOP is and why it is important.
- How COOP differs from Continuity of Government (COG).
- The roles and responsibilities of key players in COOP planning.
- Family support measures to take in case of COOP implementation.

http://training.fema.gov/EMIWeb/downloads/COOPLessonSummary.pdf

PandemicFlu.gov
Managed by the Department of Health and Human Services, this is a one-stop access to U.S. Government avian and pandemic flu information that includes planning and response guidance for a variety of outlets (Federal, state/local, individual business, school, health care, and community).

http://www.pandemicflu.gov

U.S. Office of Personnel Management: Human Capital Planning for Pandemic Influenza, Information for Agencies and Departments
This guide is designed to help Federal departments and agencies achieve two equally important goals: protecting the Federal workforce and ensuring the continuity of operations. The guide emphasizes the need to carry on the work of the Government wherever possible and through whatever means are available, including voluntary telework arrangements.

http://www.opm.gov/pandemic/

Financial

Bank of New Zealand: Business Continuity Plan (BCP) Pandemic Plan Overview
The Bank has an established BCP, which has recently been reviewed and is being further strengthened. The Bank tests its BCP preparedness on a regular basis, with Bank staff required to work from its BCP sites. In the worst-case situation of a full-scale pandemic in New Zealand, the Bank would operate with staff located at home with critical systems and activities being maintained through distributed telephone/computer systems.

http://www.rbnz.govt.nz/crisismgmt/2198851.pdf

Hospitals/Health Care Facilities

HHS Summary of Roles and Responsibilities of Health Care (Supplement 3)
Supplement 3 provides healthcare partners recommendations for developing plans to respond to an influenza pandemic. The focus is on planning during the Interpandemic Period for: pandemic influenza surveillance; decisionmaking structures for responding to a pandemic; hospital communications; education and training; patient triage; clinical evaluation and admission; facility access; managing workers; and continuation of essential medical services. In addition, it includes planning for the provision of care in non-hospital settings, including: residential care facilities; physicians' offices; private home healthcare services; emergency medical services; federally qualified health centers (FQHCs); rural health clinics; and alternative care sites.

http://www.hhs.gov/pandemicflu/plan/sup3.html

Influenza Pandemic Plan Guide for Healthcare Facilities: New Jersey Department of Health and Senior Services

This guide is intended to assist pandemic influenza planning efforts for medical provider organizations, health care systems, hospitals, long-term care facilities, community (home) health agencies, and other groups that will provide health care services as part of an influenza pandemic response. A proportion of this guide addresses the issues of how an influenza pandemic will impact services at the facility, the number of staff necessary to maintain essential services, chain of responsibility, human resource issues, and business continuity.

http://www.state.nj.us/health/flu/documents/influenza_plan.pdf

Service Continuity Planning, a Guide for Community Pharmacists (England, Wales, and Scotland)

This guidance focuses on service continuity planning within each individual pharmacy. However, community pharmacists need to consider the wider picture within their locality, such as the need to relocate to other premises, Primary Care Organization (PCO) plans, and the need to work with other contractors.

http://www.psnc.org.uk/uploaded_txt/ServiceContinuityPlanningforpharmacyguidance.pdf

Aspen Regional Health: Pandemic Plan Overview

This overview has been tailored to assist Aspen Health in meeting the responsibilities to complete the following:

- Provide the health promotion, prevention, diagnostic, treatment, rehabilitative and palliative services, supplies, equipment, and care that the regulations require it to provide.
- Resume health functions, services, programs, and operations within a reasonable time frame to enable health agents to fulfill their mission and mandate.
- Implement public health control measures to help limit the spread of disease.
- Provide information on a regional basis to protect public health and safety.
- Provide direction and advice to coordinate provision of exceptional resources to institutions, health agents, and others, and to ensure intra-regional cooperation.
- Recover Aspen Health services, functions, and infrastructure sufficiently for the health agents to resume business in an order of priority of:
  - Mission Critical Public Services—without the service, people are at risk.
  - Essential Business Functions—critical leadership and decisionmaking.
  - Priority Public Services—consequence management function related to safety.
  - Priority Business Functions—primary business support functions.

http://www.aspenrha.com/images/stories/pdf/pandemic/pandemic_overview.pdf

Pandemic Influenza COOP for Massachusetts Hospitals
This plan outlines a comprehensive approach to ensure the continuity of essential services during an influenza pandemic while ensuring the safety and well-being of employees, the emergency delegation of authority, the safekeeping of records vital to the agency and its clients, emergency acquisition of resources necessary for business resumption, and the capabilities to work at alternative work sites until normal operations can be resumed.

http://mass.gov/dph/bioterrorism/advisorygrps/word_files/hospital_coop_11_05.doc

Local Government

Metropolitan King County (Seattle) Council 2006 Pandemic COOP
This COOP contains a list of what could be expected to affect local government during a pandemic flu. It also explains the action items needed to assist operating issues for the local government of King County during a pandemic.

http://mkcclegisearch.metrokc.gov/attachments/20144.doc

Pandemic Influenza COOP Guide and Template for San Francisco City and County Agencies
The Pandemic Influenza COOP Guide and Template has been developed by the San Francisco Department of Public Health to assist city agencies think through critical issues related to pandemic influenza and create comprehensive plans to address those infrastructure needs.

http://www.sfcdcp.org/UserFiles/File/InfectiousDiseasesAtoZ/City_Agency._Pan_Flu_
Continuity_Plan.6.19.06.pdf

Santa Rosa County Pandemic Flu Plan
This plan is designed to facilitate the continuity of governmental operations in continuing to provide necessary services to the citizens of the County in the event that a pandemic strikes the Gulf Coast of Florida.

http://www.santarosa.fl.gov/emergency/documents/pandemicfluplan06.pdf

Public Health Departments

COOP Plan for Local Health Departments: MA Department of Public Health
This COOP Plan provides policy and guidance to ensure the execution of essential functions in the event that operations are threatened by a major emergency. Consolidation of planning documents into a comprehensive emergency plan is advised to enhance simplicity and ease of use. *This COOP is not specific to a pandemic COOP throughout the entire document.*

http://www.mahb.org/emergencyprep/COOP.doc

South Carolina Department of Health and Environmental Control: Pandemic Influenza Continuity of Operations Guide and Template

The pandemic influenza planning template has been developed by the South Carolina Department of Health and Environmental Control to assist county agencies in creating comprehensive pandemic influenza COOP plans. The content within the template is a launching point for developing a pandemic influenza COOP plan. It will be necessary for the agencies to refine the language to transform the template into a document that accurately represents the specific organization. Users may find that certain key issues that are important to their organization's ability to function are not addressed and may wish to add sections/subsections to the template, or choose to delete sections that are not applicable to their agency. The Annex contains information on how organizations will continue certain activities and examples and worksheets are provided to help develop this information.

http://horrycounty.redcross.org/panflu/PICOOP_Guide.doc

Appendix 2: Tabletop Exercises

This appendix contains a collection of websites that will help you in developing tabletop exercises for your organization. As with the websites for COOP planning, no one site will meet your organization's specific needs. However, drawing from a variety of websites will likely help you design an exercise that can truly test your organization's readiness. As with the COOP websites, these are organized by sector (education, government, financial, etc.).

Helpful Websites for Developing Your Tabletop Exercise

Education
http://www.tallytown.com/redcross/exercise/UniversityPandemicInfluenzaTabletopExercise-Overview.pdf
http://www.tallytown.com/redcross/exercise/UniversityPandemicInfluenzaTabletopExercise.pdf
http://edcp.org/pdf/DHMHSummaryPanFluSchoolTTX.pdf
http://www.cshema.org/resource/UNC%20System%20Pandemic%20Tabletop%20Planning%20Exercise.doc
Federal Government
http://www.hhs.gov/nvpo/pandemics/tabletopex.html
Financial
http://www.bondmarkets.com/assets/files/SIABMA_pandemicTestimony.pdf
General Operations
http://www.steadfastresponse.com
Hospitals/Health Care Facilities
http://www.nyc.gov/html/doh/downloads/pdf/bhpp/bhpp-train-hospital-toolkit.pdf
Local Government
http://www.hsph.harvard.edu/hcphp/products/exercises/HSPH-CPHP%20Avian%20&%20Pandemic%20Influenza%20Tabletop.pdf
http://www.rand.org/pubs/technical_reports/2006/RAND_TR319.pdf
http://www.nyc.gov/html/doh/downloads/pdf/bhpp/bhpp-train-city-panmod1.pdf
http://www.nyc.gov/html/doh/downloads/pdf/bhpp/bhpp-train-city-panmod2.pdf
http://www.tallytown.com/redcross/exercise/InfluenzaPandemicTabletopExercise.pdf
Public Health Departments
http://cdc.confex.com/cdc/nic2004/techprogram/session_893.htm
http://www.phppo.cdc.gov/phtn/DLSummit2005/Benton.pdf
http://www.dallascounty.org/department/hhservices/services/publichealthalert/documents/AfterActionReportFinal.pdf
http://www.idready.org/docs/DHSPanFluTableTop.pdf
http://www.liebertonline.com/doi/pdfplus/10.1089/bsp.2005.3.61

Table A2-1

Appendix 2: Tabletop Exercises

Following is a short synopsis of the websites listed in Table A2-1.

Education

University of Minnesota Pandemic Influenza Tabletop Exercise
The exercise consists of five separate scripts, each with a list of events that have occurred and data injected as appropriate. The overall goal of the exercise is to assess how the existing emergency response structure at the University of Minnesota addresses the challenges posed by pandemic influenza and how the University coordinates its response with state and local public health agencies and with Fairview University Medical Center. The exercise involves a novel H5N1 avian influenza strain that is capable of causing severe disease in humans (similar to the 1918 pandemic) and is readily transmissible through person-to-person spread. Key aspects of the exercise include the following:

- A vaccine against the novel H5N1 strain will not be available until approximately four months after the pandemic arrives in the United States.
- The scenario is assumed to be plausible and the scripts are designed to be relatively realistic, given current information about H5N1 avian influenza in Asia.
- The events unfold in the order that the scripts are presented. However, there may be days to weeks between each of the scripts and, therefore, the exercise is not intended to simulate a "real-time event."
- The scenario is designed to assess certain key decisions and issues that will need to be addressed relatively early in the course of the pandemic. Therefore, the exercise focuses on the early stages of the pandemic. Given time constraints, the exercise is not intended to cover the entire first wave of the pandemic period.

Overview:
http://www.tallytown.com/redcross/exercise/UniversityPandemicInfluenzaTabletopExercise-Overview.pdf
Script #1:
http://www.tallytown.com/redcross/exercise/UniversityPandemicInfluenzaTabletopExercise.pdf

Maryland Department of Public Health and Mental Hygiene, Summary of the Pandemic Influenza School System Tabletop Exercise
The joint school system/public health exercise was sponsored by the Maryland Department of Health and Mental Hygiene, Maryland Partnership for Prevention, and the Maryland State Department of Education.

The key findings included:

- Current local school plans do not address pandemic influenza.
- Current pandemic influenza preparedness plans do not sufficiently address school systems.
- Gaps are present in communication needed to ensure timely and effective exchange of information during an influenza pandemic.
- School systems lack specific guidance and procedures on a myriad of issues relevant to an influenza pandemic.

Recommendations included integrating pandemic influenza response plans with other local emergency preparedness efforts so that they can be regularly reviewed, developing a pandemic influenza decision matrix, and developing comprehensive communication protocols.

http://edcp.org/pdf/DHMHSummaryPanFluSchoolTTX.pdf

The University of North Carolina: Pandemic Influenza Tabletop Emergency Exercise
This is the situation manual for a tabletop exercise of the emergency preparedness of the 16-campus University of North Carolina system. This exercise focuses on a pandemic flu event that poses a severe threat to public health and safety. The overall goal of the exercise is to:

- Assess how the existing emergency response structure on campus will address the challenges posed by a pandemic influenza event.
- Assess how the campus will coordinate its response with its campus health service, area hospitals, and state and local public health agencies.
- Identify gaps and issues to be addressed in the campus response plan.
- Educate the participants about contagious disease and the unique challenges a pandemic poses to the health and well being of the university community.

http://www.cshema.org/resource/UNC%20System%20Pandemic%20Tabletop%20Planning%20Exercise.doc

Federal Government

HHS Tabletop Exercise Package
The purpose of this pandemic influenza tabletop exercise package is to provide states and local areas with tools to assist in planning and conducting tabletop exercises on the topic of pandemic influenza. Exercises serve to identify where plans may need to be refined or modified, and thus lead to strengthening preparedness. Exercises should be viewed as an integral part of planning activities.

This package includes two exercises: an overview and a surge capacity exercise, as well as other resources helpful in planning and conducting these exercises. The exercises are designed for use at the state or local level and are general enough to be useful in any area. The overview exercise addresses planning issues that will arise during the course of an influenza pandemic over an array of areas, including surveillance, vaccination, antiviral medications, communications, and emergency response. Participants for the overview exercise will include people who will be involved in planning for and responding to a pandemic, including, but not limited to, staff in the areas of public health, public information, public safety, emergency management, and health care. The surge capacity exercise focuses on medical surge capacity issues; these issues are addressed in greater depth than in the overview exercise. Participants in the surge capacity exercise will be from the same groups as for the overview exercise, but more heavily skewed toward representatives of local hospitals and emergency management services. This package is referenced by several other tabletop exercise websites and plans. It describes a few different structures, so the organization using it can choose the best approach for their own needs.

http://www.hhs.gov/nvpo/pandemics/tabletopex.html

Financial

TMBA/SIA Joint Tabletop Exercise on Industry Preparedness
The Bond Market Association and Securities Industry Association conducted a joint exercise on pandemic response issues involving fourteen of the largest securities firms. The firms were presented with an escalating pandemic scenario that focused attention on issues that would likely affect the operation of the financial markets and asked how they would respond to the changing situations. A dominant question that arose was how regulators would react in a crisis. Participants agreed regulators have been responsive and understanding in past emergencies, but there remains a concern that regulators across all markets act consistently.

http://www.bondmarkets.com/assets/files/SIABMA_pandemicTestimony.pdf

General Operations

Steadfast Response
This website offers a downloadable COOP tabletop exercise kit with a pandemic influenza scenario for general operations. The template can be used for both business and government organizations, and is claimed to have been used by Federal, state, and local players in over thirty cities.

http://www.steadfastresponse.com

Hospitals/Health Care Facilities

The New York City Department of Health and Mental Hygiene: Hospital and Primary Care Centers Tabletop Toolkit
NYC DOHMH developed this tabletop toolkit during 2004–2005 to aid hospitals in conducting exercises. The materials were tested in ten hospitals and five primary care centers in New York City and served as an important resource for staff training and a method to evaluate facility preparedness involving five biological agents, one of which is pandemic influenza. The Toolkit contents can be modified to account for the distinct geographic, patient, resource, and staffing challenges faced by individual hospitals and primary care centers. The Toolkit also includes instructions on planning, conducting, and evaluating a hospital tabletop exercise.

http://www.nyc.gov/html/doh/downloads/pdf/bhpp/bhpp-train-hospital-toolkit.pdf

Local Government

Harvard School of Public Health Center for Public Health Preparedness, Tabletop Exercise Number 1: Avian Influenza
This tabletop allows local public health officials to test their response to a major outbreak of a theoretical highly contagious and highly morbid disease. The major public health functions tested in this drill are: risk communication; isolation and quarantine procedures; and mass prophylaxis and dispensing capabilities. Additional communitywide functions tested in this drill are: risk communication; control of population movement; isolation and quarantine procedures; and protection of staff. It is recommended that exercises include representation from local public safety, local government, and major local health care providers, whenever possible, in order to integrate the community emergency response plans and facilitate cooperation.

http://www.hsph.harvard.edu/hcphp/products/exercises/HSPH-CPHP%20Avian%20&%20Pandemic%20Influenza%20Tabletop.pdf

Tabletop Exercises for Pandemic Influenza Preparedness in Local Public Health Agencies, RAND Tabletop Exercises Template
This report presents a fully customizable template for a tabletop exercise for pandemic influenza preparedness that can be used by state and local health agencies and their healthcare and governmental partners as an exercise in training, building relationships, and evaluation. The exercise relies on a "forced decision making" framework, which requires participants to make key decisions at each discussion point after they have had time to consider the scenario and the information provided to them at a specified point in "x" time. The exercise focuses on five broad issues: surveillance and epidemiology; command, control, and communications; risk communication; surge capacity; and disease prevention and control.

http://www.rand.org/pubs/technical_reports/2006/RAND_TR319.pdf

NYC Citywide Pandemic Influenza Tabletop Exercise
This exercise includes two modules used for a teleconference led by the New York City Department of Health and Mental Hygiene. Module 1 describes early pandemic activity, including vaccine production, surveillance efforts, and initial cases in localized areas of New York. Module 2 describes peak pandemic activity, providing the expected impact of the first pandemic wave, including the number of illnesses, hospital admissions, and deaths. In this phase, participants must face issues like hospital staff shortages and short supply of critical care beds and ventilators, and possibly an altered standard of care.

Module 1: http://www.nyc.gov/html/doh/downloads/pdf/bhpp/bhpp-train-city-panmod1.pdf
Module 2: http://www.nyc.gov/html/doh/downloads/pdf/bhpp/bhpp-train-city-panmod2.pdf

Leon County Health Department Influenza Pandemic Tabletop Exercise
This exercise focuses on communication, emergency response coordination, resource integration, problem identification, and resolution. This exercise is meant to focus on the overall response and decisionmaking process and is not a test of detailed response procedures. It is divided into three modules: incubation, intensification, and escalation. The objectives are:

- Exercise the local and regional decisionmaking process and identify areas needing refinements. Identify key actions to be taken and by whom.
- Review local, state, and Federal operations for area access control and possible quarantine issues resulting from an epidemiological incident.
- Examine the local interface among city, county, state, and Federal agencies in the conduct of crisis and consequence management activities. Examine local, state, and Federal interactions with the private and public sector during the threat or actual occurrence of an epidemiological incident.
- Discuss options to provide timely information to the population and assist in minimizing chaos. Review plans to preclude dissemination of conflicting data. Assess the adequacy of local plans for interface with and use of media resources. Discuss how media will be coordinated when state and Federal agencies are involved.
- Review the local medical, emergency medical transport, and public health department capabilities to recognize, identify, monitor, and respond to an incident involving an influenza pandemic.

http://www.tallytown.com/redcross/exercise/InfluenzaPandemicTabletopExercise.pdf

Public Health Departments

CDC Session: Advancing Pandemic Influenza Planning through Tabletop Exercises
This workshop describes the experiences of Massachusetts, Maryland, and Minnesota in planning and conducting pandemic influenza tabletop exercises. Participants should be able to identify key steps in planning and conducting a tabletop exercise and understand how exercises can improve the planning process.

http://cdc.confex.com/cdc/nic2004/techprogram/session_893.htm

California Department of Health Services
This presentation on using live satellite broadcast to prepare for pandemic influenza offers background information on avian influenza and detailed advice on how to plan a broadcast and tabletop exercise. The exercise objectives are to familiarize individuals with their local jurisdiction's pandemic influenza plan and to practice two of the ten deliverables that should be included in a pandemic influenza plan. These deliverables include:
- Draft possible key messages and use them to write a press release about pandemic influenza in general *before* a local outbreak has occurred.
- Identify agency partners, as well as other stakeholders, who would be involved in two of the listed response activities, and list their respective roles and responsibilities.
- Test your organization's emergency response command and communication structure by drawing a schematic of the response structure and information flow, or a call-down tree, to activate emergency response plan.
- Draft a checklist, step-by-step plan, or flowchart on the type of communication channels that will be used, how they will be used, and the populations that the channels will reach.

http://www.phppo.cdc.gov/phtn/DLSummit2005/Benton.pdf

Dallas County Health and Human Services (DCHHS), Avian Flu Pandemic Tabletop Exercise After Action Report
This exercise allowed participants to discuss issues in a logical sequence within a hypothetical scenario. The response was divided into three phases: identification and notification, public health emergency, and response efforts. Future recommendations included:

- Local, state, and private sector partners should continue to review and evaluate their procedures for an effective multi-agency response during a pandemic event.
- Additional private sector organizations need to participate and partner with DCHHS in future exercises and symposiums to develop stronger community involvement.
- For hospitals: institute regional hospital collaboration, create a framework for allocation of limited medical resources, and revise pandemic preparedness guidance for hospitals.

The purpose of this exercise was to facilitate understanding of concepts, identify strengths and shortfalls, and educate key partner organizations, to include the private sector, in pandemic response and recovery requirements. It also provided participants an opportunity to evaluate current response concepts, plans, and capabilities for a community-wide response to a large-scale, public health emergency that was health based, not disaster based.

http://www.dallascounty.org/department/hhservices/services/publichealthalert/documents/AfterActionReportFinal.pdf

California Division of Communicable Disease Control (DCDC), Pandemic Influenza Tabletop Exercise
This DCDC problem-solving tabletop exercise presented four different scenarios that required prompt responses in order to orient DCDC participants to the draft pandemic response plan:

- Identify how key response measures will be implemented.
- Identify gaps and vulnerabilities in DCDC pandemic influenza preparedness.
- Make specific recommendations for plan revisions.
- Promote inter-program collaboration and coordination.

The exercise addresses command and control, operations/planning section functions, communications section functions, logistic section functions, and miscellaneous topics.

http://www.idready.org/docs/DHSPanFluTableTop.pdf

Maryland Department of Health and Mental Hygiene, Pandemic Influenza Preparedness in Maryland: Improving Readiness through a Tabletop Exercise
During the tabletop exercise meant to test the Maryland Pandemic Influenza Preparedness Plan, participants were presented with nine different fictitious scripts encompassing a single scenario. They were asked to respond to the information presented in each script, discuss organization-specific questions posed by the exercise facilitator, and make decisions regarding action steps that their organization would take in response to the various issues raised. The exercise identified a number of important gaps that need to be addressed, including: additional surge capacity specific to a pandemic; greater understanding of the realities and implications of pandemic influenza among elected officials and decision makers; coordination of pandemic influenza planning with the existing emergency response infrastructure coupled with additional training in incident command; further steps to make several aspects of the Maryland Pandemic Influenza Preparedness Plan operational; and additional Federal guidance.

http://www.liebertonline.com/doi/pdfplus/10.1089/bsp.2005.3.61

www.ingramcontent.com/pod-product-compliance
Lightning Source LLC
Chambersburg PA
CBHW081601170526
45166CB00009B/2781